Lecture Notes on Nephrology

D.B. Evans

MB, BCh, FRCP
Consultant Physician
Renal Unit
Addenbrooke's Hospital
Cambridge
Associate Lecturer in Medicine to
The University of Cambridge

AND

R.G. Henderson

MD, MRCP
Consultant Physician
Hinchingbrooke Hospital
Huntingdon
and to the Renal Unit
Addenbrooke's Hospital
Associate Lecturer in Medicine to
The University of Cambridge

BLACKWELL
SCIENTIFIC PUBLICATIONS
OXFORD LONDON EDINBURGH
BOSTON PALO ALTO MELBOURNE

© 1985 by
Blackwell Scientific Publications
Editorial offices:
Osney Mead, Oxford, OX2 0EL
8 John Street, London, WC1N 2ES
23 Ainslie Place, Edinburgh,
  EH3 6AJ
52 Beacon Street, Boston
  Massachusetts 02108, USA
706 Cowper Street, Palo Alto
  California 94301, USA
107 Barry Street, Carlton
  Victoria 3053, Australia

First published 1985

Set by Butler & Tanner Ltd, Frome
Printed and bound in Great Britain
by Billing & Sons Ltd, Worcester

DISTRIBUTORS

USA
  Blackwell Mosby Book
    Distributors
  11830 Westline Industrial Drive
  St Louis, Missouri 63141

Canada
  Blackwell Mosby Book
    Distributors
  120 Melford Drive, Scarborough
  Ontario, M1B 2X4

Australia
  Blackwell Scientific Book
    Distributors
  31 Advantage Road, Highett
  Victoria 3190

British Library
Cataloguing in Publication Data

Evans, D.B.
  Lecture notes on nephrology.
  1. Kidneys—Diseases
  I. Title   II. Henderson, R.G.
  616.6′1   RC902

ISBN 0-632-00283-2

Contents

Preface

In the past few years there has been a proliferation of short textbooks in various specialities including nephrology, so that students are spoilt for choice. How then does one choose the right book? As medical curricula expand, students are expected to assimilate more and more facts. Therefore, condensation of what is important without dressing it up to appear complicated would seem to us to be of prime importance. This is what we have tried to do in this edition of *Lecture Notes on Nephrology*. This is not intended to be a comprehensive textbook but a list of suggested Further Reading is included to satisfy those inclined to more profound enquiry.

We would like to acknowledge the help and encouragement given by our wives during the lengthy gestation of this book, the expert secretarial help from Mrs J. Small who typed the countless proofs and the patience of Mr Peter Saugman of Blackwell Scientific Publications.

Finally, we are grateful for the help and forebearance of our past teachers, colleagues, nursing colleagues and patients, without which we would not have been able even to attempt to write this book.

D.B. Evans
R.G. Henderson

Chapter 1
History Taking and Examination in Renal Disease

INTRODUCTION

Occasionally a patient may give a brief history which by its very nature will lead to a rapid diagnosis. A sore throat followed two weeks later by oliguria may well lead to the correct diagnosis of acute glomerulonephritis, whilst a history of colicky loin pain extending to the testicle followed later by the passage of a stone in the urine leaves no doubt as to the diagnosis. Similarly, examination may provide all the clues necessary to make a diagnosis but in general this is unusual. More often the patient will have suffered a chronic illness extending over many years sometimes from childhood so that aetiological clues will have to be carefully sought. The presence of significant renal disease not yet severe enough to cause symptoms may well be missed unless the urine is tested. This simple investigation should *always* be performed as part of the physical examination and failure to do so is a serious error.

Diagnostic features of the history and examination will be found in the relevant sections of this book but a few points are worth emphasizing.

HISTORY

1 Since many disease processes affecting the kidneys are chronic the past and present medical histories often merge.

2 In early childhood, persistent enuresis, intermittent fevers, dysuria, loin or abdominal pain, vomiting and episodes of non-specific ill-health may all point towards recurrent urinary infections which may lead to scarring and impairment of kidney growth.

3 Pregnancy is a good test of renal function and enquiry should be made whether pregnancies were complicated by urinary infection, hypertension, or ankle swelling.

4 Medical examinations performed for insurance purposes or on

1

entry or discharge from the services may also provide a clue as to the presence of hypertension or proteinuria.

5   A past history of acute glomerulonephritis may be elicited. The patient may recall an illness characterized by swelling of the face and ankles which led to a long period of absence from school and considerable bed rest.

6   A history of loin pain is important:

(a)   where it occurs during micturition spreading from the suprapubic region up to one or other of the loins, which would suggest reflux nephropathy;

(b)   starting in the loin area and radiating down to the testicle and associated with haematuria and perhaps grit or gravel in the urine when a diagnosis of renal calculus is likely;

(c)   a non-specific loin pain particularly occurring at periods of high fluid intake and associated with a normal urinary sediment might suggest the diagnosis of hydronephrosis;

(d)   progressively worse loin pain associated with malaise and weight loss may indicate a renal tumour.

7   Abnormal bladder function should be sought since this may predispose to infection, calculus formation and reflux. Enquiries should be made about initiation of micturition, strength of stream and terminal dribbling. The capacity to pass a significant amount of urine a few minutes after micturition would suggest either ureteric reflux, a bladder diverticulum or incomplete emptying of the bladder.

8   Proteinuria may be suggested by frothy urine and if this is severe enough to cause hypoalbuminaemia then ankle oedema may occur.

9   Renal involvement leads to a loss of concentrating ability early on and this will manifest itself as nocturnal frequency.

10   Enquiry should be made into all systems since renal involvement may be part of a multisystem disease such as diabetes mellitus, multiple myeloma, amyloidosis or tuberculosis.

11   The family history is important. Where there is a history of renal failure then the possibility of polycystic disease, Alport's syndrome etc. should be considered. A knowledge of genetics will provide additional information, for when renal disease is associated with deafness, Alport's syndrome is very likely, whereas a family history of renal calculi might suggest renal tubular acidosis, cystinosis, oxaluria, etc.

12   A drug history is nowadays most important. Certain agents are directly nephrotoxic, e.g. cephaloridine, gentamicin, while others may, in certain individuals, cause an acute interstitial nephropathy, e.g. antipyretics and thiazide diuretics. It is particularly important where acute renal failure has developed in hospital to find out what drugs the patient has received for they may be responsible for the problems. Analgesic abuse should be sought in every patient presenting with chronic renal failure. It is often useless to ask the patient directly whether he has been taking analgesics since this may lead to a denial but rather, the patient should be asked whether he has suffered from any chronic pain and whether he has bought medication from the chemist for this. The length of time that a hundred tablets would last the patient usually gives a reasonable guide to ingestion.

13 Occupational history is important, for exposure to substances such as lead, dry cleaning fluids, etc., can lead to renal damage. There is increasing evidence that exposure to hydrocarbons in all sorts of occupations may be associated with an increased incidence of glomerulonephritis.

EXAMINATION

In terms of physical signs renal disease is rather disappointing compared with diseases affecting the chest or cardiovascular systems. However, the following are important.

1 Occasionally the patient will have all the clinical signs of one of the syndromes such as chronic renal failure (see p. 125) or the nephrotic syndrome (see p. 74).

2 The kidneys should be palpated, for if one or both are palpable, a diagnosis of polycystic disease, hydronephrosis, tumour, etc., is likely.

3 The presence of an enlarged bladder would suggest lower urinary obstruction. If of long standing, this is likely to lead to infection, stone formation and renal impairment.

4 Pyrexia in the presence of tenderness over the bladder or the kidneys suggests infection and perhaps abscess formation.

5 The blood pressure should always be measured both lying and standing and an assessment should be made of the patient's fluid status. If the blood pressure is raised, then its effect upon target organs particularly the fundi and heart, should be sought.

6 Finally, evidence of multisystem disease should be looked for.

URINE EXAMINATION

This is mandatory in all patients whatever their complaint. Stick
testing will reveal the presence of protein, blood and glucose in a
semi-quantitative manner. Additional information may be gleaned
by urine microscopy but, unfortunately, this has now been relegated
to the laboratory from the ward side rooms. Some reagent sticks
contain nitrite-detecting reagents which, in the presence of certain
bacteria, convert the nitrate derived from metabolites into nitrite
thereby suggesting urinary infection. Unfortunately this test lacks
sensitivity and its use may lead to urinary infections being missed.
Whenever a suspicion of urinary pathology is raised a urine sample
should be submitted to the laboratory for microscopy and culture.

Chapter 2
Anatomy

The kidneys are paired organs situated high in the retroperitoneal regions of the abdomen and in relation to the 10th, 11th and 12th ribs. The right kidney lies slightly lower than the left (Fig. 2.1). Each measures approximately 12–14 cms in length when fully grown and weighs about 150 g (Fig. 2.1). Normally the blood supply via the renal arteries comes direct from the aorta and the renal veins drain into the inferior vena cava. Urine collects in the renal pelvis which leads via the ureters to the bladder.

The surface of each kidney is smooth and is a purplish-brown colour. It has a thin capsule.

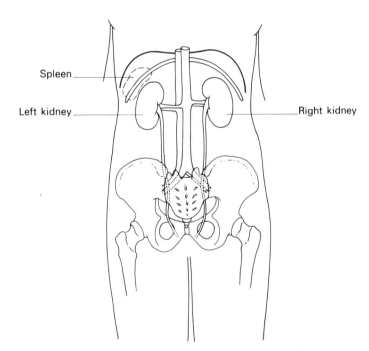

Fig. 2.1 The anatomical position of the kidneys (posterior view).

The cut surface of the kidney shows clearly defined structures— a cortex and medulla, pyramids, calyces and pelvis. Between each pyramid lie the columns of Bertini.

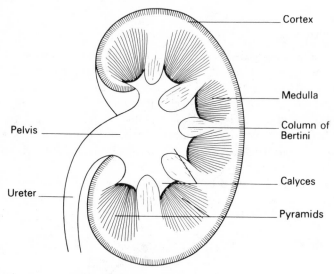

Fig. 2.2 A section through the normal kidney.

BLOOD SUPPLY

The kidney may be supplied by a single artery or by multiple arteries. These, in turn, may branch before entering the hilar structures. Inside the kidney they divide to form interlobar arteries which traverse the renal medulla as far as the corticomedullary junction. Arcuate arteries are then formed from the interlobar arteries and these run parallel to the outer surface of the kidney and at right angles to the interlobars at the corticomedullary junction (Fig. 2.3). From the arcuate arteries rise the interlobular arteries which pass into the cortex and from which the afferent glomerular arterioles arise. From the efferent glomerular arterioles emerges the bed of peritubular capillaries which either empties into peritubular venules or plunges alongside the loops of Henle into the medulla to form the vasa recta. They eventually drain into the venous system which follows anatomically the arterial system.

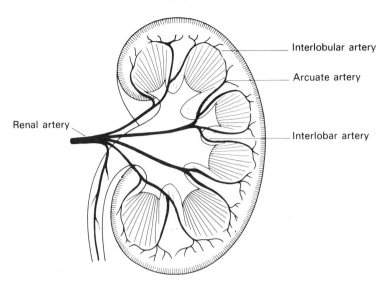

Fig. 2.3 Arterial supply to the kidney.

THE NEPHRON

Each kidney is composed of approximately 1 million functional units, known as nephrons. It is in these that blood is filtered and urine elaborated (Fig. 2.4).

Outer cortical nephrons have no loops of Henle and are concerned mainly with sodium regulation.

Inner cortical nephrons have long loops and are mainly concerned with the process of urinary concentration.

The nephrons are packed closely together in the kidney in such a way that adjacent structures tend to influence each other's function.

The structure and function of every component of the nephron is highly specialized.

The glomerulus

Glomerular capillaries arise from the afferent arteriole and terminate in the efferent arteriole. They develop *in situ* by differentiation of mesenchymal cells, situated in close proximity to the beginning of the tubular duct, culminating in an intricate branching network indenting Bowman's capsule (Fig. 2.5).

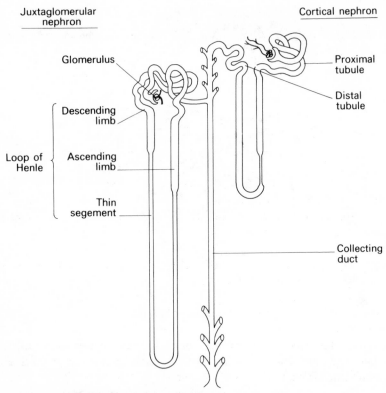

Fig. 2.4 The structure of the nephron.

The afferent arteriolar wall is a muscular structure. Those at the corticomedullary junction also possess cells which contain electron-dense granules and rough endoplasmic reticulum. These are the juxtaglomerular cells and they are thought to be the source of renin and possibly also of a sodium-regulating hormone.

The efferent arteriole is slightly narrower than the afferent and also has smooth muscle fibres in its wall.

Glomerular capillaries

They are composed of three layers—epithelium, basement membrane and endothelium (Fig. 2.6). In the central area of the glomerular tuft are the mesangium-containing cells.

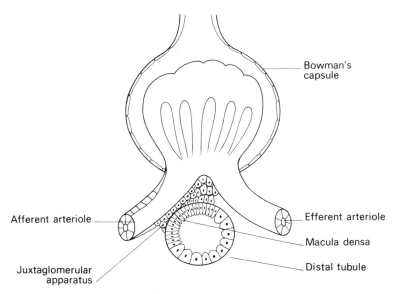

Fig. 2.5   The composition of the glomerulus.

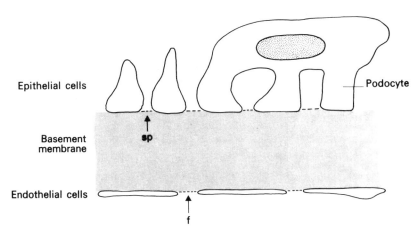

Fig. 2.6   The three layers of the glomerular capillary.

Endothelial cells are extensions of the afferent arteriolar endothelium. Numerous fenestrations (f) are present in them and these are bridged over by a thin diaphragm.

Basement membrane lies between endothelial and epithelial cells and is probably a homogeneous structure though a central denser region has been described. Its structure is ill defined but many people have suggested that it is composed of short delicate filaments arranged in an irregular meshwork similar to filter paper.

The epithelium is continuous with the parietal layer of Bowman's capsule. Each mature cell has a nucleus and long cell processes called podocytes (foot processes) which, in turn, are subdivided into smaller outgrowths or pedicels which interdigitate with each other and with similar pedicels from adjacent epithelial cells. The spaces between the pedicels are known as slit pores (sp) which are bridged by a thin filamentous membrane with a central thickening.

Mesangial cells are centrally situated in the glomerular tuft and are surrounded by matrix. They are considered to be of mesenchymal origin and when required they may develop into endothelial cells and, furthermore, may be capable of generating new basement membrane material. In some situations they may have phagocytic properties.

Proximal convoluted tubule is situated in the cortex. The epithelium is cuboidal and one layer deep. It has large basal nuclei—cell boundaries are irregular and interdigitated with boundaries of adjacent cells. The luminal surface has a brush border. The basal cell surface has many infoldings and high ATPase activity has been found in these regions. In the organ cells a Golgi zone surrounds the nucleus and there are numerous mitochondria.

The thin segment of Henle's loop is very short or absent in outer cortical nephrons. In juxtamedullary nephrons the loop descends into the medulla. The diameter is much less than that of the proximal tubule. Cells are flat and squamous and are star fish shaped; only a few mitochondria are present. Luminal surfaces have few short microvilli.

Distal tubule cells are cuboidal. Cytoplasma contains abundant rod-like mitochondria—mainly in the basal two-thirds of the cells and ribosomes. The nuclei are near the apex of the cell. The luminal surface has short microvilli. The apices of the cells are pervaded by numerous tiny vesicles. The basal surfaces have many clefts (Fig. 2.7).

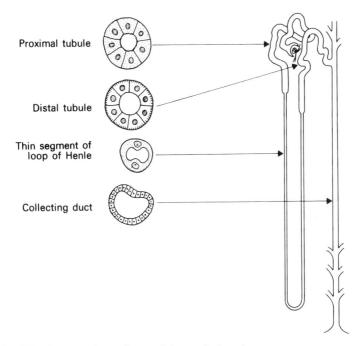

Proximal tubule

Distal tubule

Thin segment of loop of Henle

Collecting duct

Fig. 2.7   Cross-sections of part of the cortical nephron.

Macula densa.   When the distal tubule returns to the vicinity of its own glomerulus it makes a short tangiential contact with the afferent arteriole. At that point the tubular cells become narrow and the nuclei are densely crowded together. Mitochondria are scarce and round in shape (Fig. 2.5).

Collecting tubules contain cuboidal cells with only a few organelles. The luminal surface has short, coarse microvilli. The basal surface is smooth.

Pelvis, ureter and bladder have muscular walls which are lined by transitional epithelium.

EMBRYOLOGY

The basic elements of the kidney are derived from the mesoderm of the intermediate cell mass and the endoderm of the cloaca.

When the embryo is 2.5 mm long two longitudinal ducts develop lateral to the mesodermal cell mass on each side of the body and grow down to reach the cloaca. The pronephros and mesonephros develop in association with this (the Wolffian) duct. The pronephros appears early but regresses rapidly and the mesonephros then develops into a primitive excretory organ. It also later undergoes atrophy and the metanephros (permanent kidney) develops. The mesonephros is represented in the male by the excretory apparatus of the testes and in the female as a vestigial remnant in the broad ligament.

The excretory portion of the permanent kidney eventually develops from the fusion of the metanephric ducts and the collecting ducts from the ureteric bud.

The kidneys in the embryo develop opposite the vertebra L3 but as the embryo elongates they appear to move in a cranial direction to be eventually opposite D12 to L2. They also rotate through 90° so that their pelves lie medially.

Chapter 3
Renal Function

The passage of blood through the glomerular capillaries of the kidneys filters approximately 170 litres of almost protein-free fluid which has the same solute concentrations as plasma. During the course of the filtrate through the nephrons, all but 1–2 litres of water are reabsorbed along with many solutes. At the same time certain substances are added to the fluid by secretion from the tubular cells. In this way the kidneys behave as organs of excretion and of conservation. In addition they have certain endocrine functions (see below).

GLOMERULAR FILTRATION

The glomerular capillary bed is unique for it is situated between two muscular blood vessels—the afferent and efferent arterioles. The process of filtration is passive and depends upon the hydrostatic pressure of the blood within the capillary and upon the permeability of the capillary membrane. The pressure outside the capillary wall and the oncotic pressure of plasma may play a small part in the process.

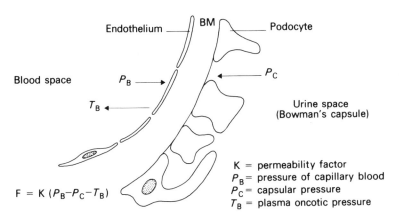

$$F = K (P_B - P_C - T_B)$$

K = permeability factor
P_B = pressure of capillary blood
P_C = capsular pressure
T_B = plasma oncotic pressure

Regulation of glomerular filtration

1 The pressure of blood in the capillaries depends on the tone in the walls of the afferent and efferent arterioles and is controlled by the renal nerves and the distensibility of the arteriolar walls (innervated kidneys).

2 The permeability of the capillary wall depends upon the area of functioning capillary tissue.

3 Capsular fluid pressure is not important except when tubular obstruction occurs.

4 Plasma protein oncotic pressure can rise to significant levels when the rate of filtration is high.

Measurement of GFR.

GFR (glomerular filtration rate) for any substance under study is defined as the volume of blood passing through the glomeruli per minute that is completely cleared of the substance.

It can be derived from the equation $GFR = U_x V/P_x$ where U_x is urinary concentration of x, V the minute volume and P_x the plasma concentration of x. The normal average GFR for a man is ~ 125 ml min^{-1}, for a woman ~ 110 ml min^{-1}.

To measure GFR accurately a substance which is neither reabsorbed nor secreted by the tubular cells must be used.

1 The starch-like polymer of fructose, inulin, is the only substance that fulfils these criteria but for practical purposes, routine inulin clearances are not very practical, for i.v. constant infusion and bladder catherization are necessary. Furthermore, a special laboratory assay has to be set up.

2 Endogeneous creatinine clearance is a more practical investigation (*vide infra*), but as creatinine is secreted by renal tubular cells it overestimates the GFR.

3 Radioactively labelled substances such as Vit B_{12}, and Ethylenediamine tetra-acetic acid (EDTA) can also be used for GFR estimation.

TUBULAR FUNCTION

The renal tubules are complex structures whose various functions contribute to the maintenance of the constancy of the 'internal environment' of the body's cells:

Tubular reabsorption—Passive (down a concentration gradient—
                                no energy required)
                              Active (against a concentration gradient
                                therefore energy required)
Tubular secretion
Urinary concentration
Regulation of salt and water excretion
Acid-base control

Passive reabsorption

Approximately 60–80% of filtered fluid is passively reabsorbed from
the proximal tubules along with solutes such as urea and potassium
secondary to the active reabsorption of sodium. Urea reabsorption
varies inversely with the rate of urine flow.

Active reabsorption

1 *Sodium.* This is the most actively reabsorbed substance from the
glomerular filtrate. Approximately 1 kg of salt is filtered by the
glomeruli per day and 60–80% of this is reabsorbed in the proximal
tubule. More energy is expended by the kidney in achieving this than
in any other of its functions.

2 *Glucose.* This is completely filtered and is normally reabsorbed
completely in the proximal tubules against a concentration gradient.

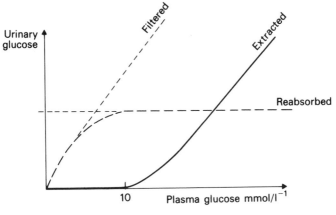

$$T_{mg} = C_{in} \times Pg - Ug \times V$$

If the blood glucose level is progressively increased, at a critical point, glucose will appear in the urine. Further increases in plasma glucose cause a proportionate rise in urinary glucose.

The critical point is reached when the tubules are reabsorbing glucose at their maximal capacity—this is known as the tubular maximal reabsorptive capacity for glucose, T_{MG}. It can be derived from the equation:

$$U_G V = C_{IN} \times P_G - T_{MG}$$

where U_G is urine glucose, V is minute volume, C_{IN} is inulin clearance, P_G is plasma glucose. The normal T_{MG} for males is 375 mg min^{-1} (21 mmol min^{-1}) and for females is 300 mg min^{-1} (16.6 mmol min^{-1}).

Other sugars seem to be handled in a similar way.

3 *Amino acids.* Only traces if these substances are present in urine normally. Groups of amino acids such as lysine, arginine and histidine have their own transport mechanisms.

4 *Phosphate.* The transport mechanism is probably inhibited by parathyroid hormone.

5 *Urates.* Transport may be blocked by a wide variety of agents, e.g. probenecid.

Tubular secretion

Substances such as potassium, hydrogen ions and ammonia are secreted into the tubular fluid from the cells. Many other substances that are not normally present in the blood are secreted, e.g. paraminohippurate (PAH), penicillin, diodrast, phenol red, thiazides, etc.

PAH is a substance that is almost completely excreted by filtration and tubular excretion and, therefore, can be used as a measure of renal plasma flow (RPF).

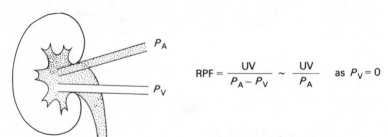

$$RPF = \frac{UV}{P_A - P_V} \sim \frac{UV}{P_A} \quad \text{as } P_V = 0$$

The normal value for RPF by this method is $600 \, \text{ml} \, \text{min}^{-1}$. The *filtration fraction* can thus be derived from

$$\frac{\text{GFR}}{\text{RPF}} = \frac{125}{600} = 0.2.$$

Urinary concentration

Nephrons whose glomeruli are situated in the inner cortex and juxtamedullary regions possess long loops of Henle that plunge into the renal medulla and return to the cortex as the distal tubule before entering the collecting ducts. Accompanying these loops are the long blood vessels or vasa recta, derived from the efferent arterioles. The vasa recta, loops of Henle and the collecting ducts are closely packed and surrounded by the interstitial fluid, so that biochemical changes in one structure are rapidly reflected in its neighbours.

As tubular fluid enters the descending portion of Henle's loop water is reabsorbed and sodium enters the tubule so that the fluid

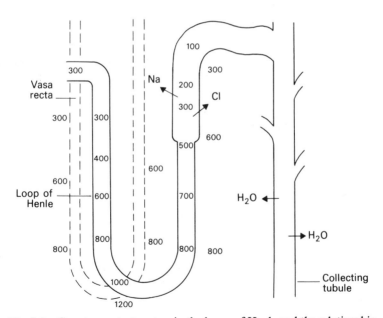

Fig. 3.1 Counter current system in the loops of Henle and the relationship to the vasa recta and collecting tubule.

becomes increasingly hypertonic as it approaches the bottom of the loop. In the ascending limb sodium and chloride are actively pumped out into the adjacent interstitial fluid, the interstitium thereby becoming hypertonic. The osmolality in the deeper parts of the medulla may increase to about 1400 mos mol kg^{-1}.

When the tubular fluid enters the distal tubule, it is hypotonic to plasma, but it rapidly equilibrates with the plasma and the final regulation of sodium, potassium and hydrogen ions takes place (Fig. 3.1). As the urine flows down the collecting ducts, its final concentration is determined by the osmotic gradient in the medulla and by the influence of antidiuretic hormone (ADH). The presence of ADH renders the tubule permeable to water so that osmotic reabsorption of water into the medullary interstitium occurs, resulting in urine osmolality approaching that of the medulla. In the absence of ADH as in diabetes insipidus (DI) the collecting duct cells remain impervious to water so that the distal tubular fluid emerges virtually unchanged.

ADH (antidiuretic hormone)

This substance is produced in the supraoptic nuclei of the hypothalamus and is transported to the posterior pituitary where it is stored, to be released when vascular osmoreceptors are stimulated by increased plasma osmolality or hypovolaemia occurs. These stimuli lead to the release of ADH resulting in changes in the permeability of the collecting duct as described above. Pain, fear, trauma, smoking and drugs can also increase the release of ADH by stimulating the central coordinating mechanism in the hypothalamus.

Sodium regulation

1 Changes in the volume of extracellular fluid plays an important role in the regulation of proximal tubular sodium reabsorption (e.g. a fall in perfusion leads to increased sodium reabsorption).

2 The glomerular filtration rate also has an influence on sodium excretion by varying the amount of sodium filtered by the glomerulus and entering the proximal tubules (Fig. 3.2).

3 The final control of sodium excretion depends on the function of the distal tubule where sodium is reabsorbed in exchange for

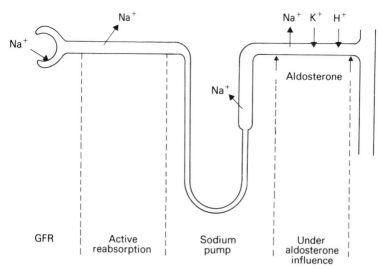

Fig. 3.2 Sodium excretion in the nephron.

potassium and hydrogen ions. The main influence seems to be the mineralocorticoid aldosterone via the renin-angiotensin system.

Evidence for a natriuretic hormone which increases sodium excretion in response to isotonic fluid loading, but independent of GFR and aldosterone, is now very strong but the mode of action of this substance is not yet fully understood.

Diuretics of various types will primarily increase sodium excretion and many of them increase potassium excretion. Thiazides and mercurial diuretics inhibit sodium transport in proximal tubules and the thiazides are weak carbonic anhydrase inhibitors. Acetazolamide is a carbonic anhydrase (CA) inhibitor but is only a very mild diuretic. The loop diuretics such as frusemide and bumetanide inhibit sodium and chloride reabsorption in the ascending limb of Henle's loop and aldosterone antagonists increase distal tubular sodium excretion in exchange for potassium (and H^+).

Osmotic diuretics, by virtue of their relative impermeability retain fluid within the tubular lumen with resulting increased rate of flow and sodium excretion.

Potassium excretion

Potassium is both reabsorbed and secreted in the tubules so that only approximately 15% of filtered potassium is excreted in urine. 60–80% of filtered K^+ is reabsorbed in the proximal tubule by a passive process but it is probably reabsorbed actively in the ascending limb of Henle's loop. Later K or H^+ may exchange for Na^+ in the distal tubule under the influence of aldosterone and metabolic alkalosis, e.g. in pyloric stenosis.

Acid-base regulation

Acid is produced continuously in the body as a result of metabolic processes, e.g. —S—S- containing amino acids get converted to sulphuric acid, protein breakdown produces phosphoric acid, etc., so that the kidney is called upon to dispose of up to 40–80 mmol of hydrogen ions per day though this could be much greater in such situations as diabetic ketoacidosis.

As these acids cannot exist in their free state in the body, they are buffered. The most abundant substance available is bicarbonate but lower down the nephron phosphate and other buffers are present:

$$H^+A^- + NaHCO_3 \rightleftharpoons Na^+A^- + H_2CO_3 \overset{ca}{\rightleftharpoons} H_2O + CO_2\uparrow$$

so that 1 mmol of acid is replaced by 1 mmol of bicarbonate. Conservation of bicarbonate, however, must take place otherwise body stores would be rapidly depleted. This can be achieved in the following ways:

1 Bicarbonate reabsorption occurs from proximal tubular fluid. H^+ is excreted in exchange for Na^+.

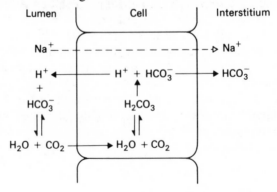

2 Excretion of H^+ as titratable acid and as NH_4^+ in exchange for bicarbonate lower down the nephron.

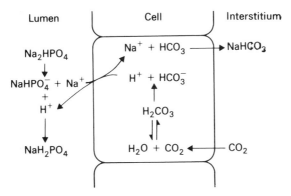

$NaHCO_3$ is reabsorbed in exchange for H^+ in the form of titratable acid NaH_2PO_4.

3 Ammonia is produced in tubular cells from deamination of amino acids, e.g. glutamine. It is lipid soluble and diffuses easily through the cell membrane into the tubular lumen where it combines with H^+ to produce NH_4^+ salts, e.g. $2NH_4HCO_3 + Na_2SO_4 \rightarrow 2NaHCO_3 + (NH_4)_2SO_4$.

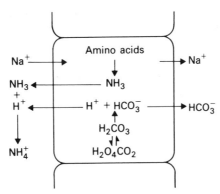

If hypokalaemia occurs, potassium will be reabsorbed in exchange for hydrogen ions. Increased bicarbonate generation occurs producing an alkalosis but the urine becomes acid.

RENIN PRODUCTION

Renin is produced by granules in the wall of the afferent arteriole of the juxtaglomerular (JG) apparatus in response to changes in sodium excretion, blood volume and to renal ischaemia. Renin reacts with a plasma substrate producing a decapeptide angiotensin I, which, in turn, is split by a converting enzyme in the lungs to an active octapeptide angiotensin II.

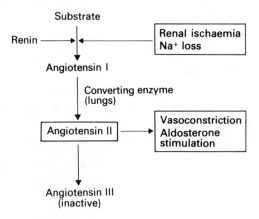

Angiotensin II is a very powerful vasoconstrictor and is probably responsible for cases of malignant hypertension of renovascular origin and in patients with renal ischaemia due to chronic renal diseases. It is also the main stimulus to the secretion of aldosterone by the adrenal cortex which it can achieve without necessarily raising the blood pressure. Under normal conditions tubular sodium retention via aldosterone will result in the inhibition of renin secretion after restoration of ECF volume to normal.

ERYTHROPOIETIN PRODUCTION

This hormone produced by the kidney stimulates erythrocyte production and is produced in excess in certain renal cystic conditions and by renal tumours. Anaemia and hypoxia will stimulate erythropoietin production and its absence in renal failure and in nephrectomized patients leads to chronic (haematinic resistant) anaemia.

Small amounts may be produced extrarenally. Assay of this substance is difficult and therapeutically it is not yet available.

NATRIURETIC HORMONE

A short-lived substance released by the kidney to stimulate sodium excretion in response to iso-osmolar fluid loading has been suspected for many years. Its presence is now certain but its chemical structure is disputed.

METABOLISM OF VITAMIN D

The elaboration of some of the active constituents of vitamin D has been shown to occur in the kidney. The hydroxylation of 25 hydroxycholecalciferol (HCC) in the 1 position to produce 1,25 dihydroxycholecalciferol (DHCC) has been established and other analogues may also be synthesized in this way.

Chapter 4
Tests of Renal Function

Detailed analyses of various aspects of renal function are tedious and are neither available nor practical in the setting of routine clinical practice. The more sophisticated tests of function will, therefore, not be discussed in this section.

The following basic investigations are those most relevant to nephrological practice and should be available in most clinical laboratories. However, one must appreciate that the degree of accuracy of many of these may not be of the highest order but should be weighed against their availability, convenience and expense.

URINALYSIS

The method of collection and its subsequent handling are most important if maximum information is to be gained. A clean catch specimen should be obtained and the urine should be collected in a clean container. The container should be sterile if bacteriological culture is contemplated. The fresh urine should be examined microscopically for cells, organisms, casts and crystals. Delay in performing this important investigation may result in the disappearance of cells and casts and the proliferation of bacteria and amorphous deposits. Tests for protein and glucose should always be performed.

Proteinuria

Protein can be detected by any of the following methods:
1 Boiling in a test tube after acidification with dilute acetic acid.
2 Addition of sulphosalicylic acid.
3 A test stick coated with bromophenol blue.
These are qualitative tests but will detect trace amounts of protein down to a concentration of 10–20 mg dl^{-1}. A quantitative estimation of proteinuria should then be performed on a 24-hour collection of urine in the laboratory. Constant proteinuria should always be con-

sidered seriously for it usually represents renal damage. The converse, however, is not always true.

Bence Jones proteinuria occurs in some forms of myelomatosis—the molecules are small light chains and are easily passed through the glomerular membrane.

It can be detected by heating the urine to 70°C when it precipitates. If heating is continued, the deposit will clear. Nowadays specific antisera are used to characterize them.

Tubular proteinuria. Tubular proteins $-\beta_1$ microglobulin, orosomucoid, Tam Horsfall protein, etc., are secreted by the tubular cells in association with certain tubular abnormalities and can be detected by special electrophoretic techniques.

Protein Selectivity Index. This is obtained by comparing the clearance rates of large and small proteins by the kidney. Usually albumin or transferrin clearance and IgG clearance are used for the purpose.

Simultaneous plasma and urine samples need to be taken for this test. A timed urine volume is not necessary. An index of less than 0.2 indicates a selective proteinuria. If greater than 0.2 it is considered to be non-selective, i.e. a relatively large amount of high molecular weight protein is being excreted.

The value of this test is mainly in children where a high degree of selectivity correlates well with minimal change glomerulonephritis. In adults it is unreliable.

Urine microscopy

Normal urine contains very occasional red cells, white cells, hyaline casts and squamous cells. No bacteria should be seen.

The presence of excess erythrocytes, leucocytes or casts is abnormal. The appearance of crystals may also be important.

Dense granular casts are composed of immunoglobulins. Cellular casts may contain red or white cells. Fatty cases may be excreted in the nephrotic syndrome.

Glomerular filtration rate (standardize to body surface area of 1.73 m²)

1 Urea clearance is no longer measured.

2 Creatinine clearance is the most commonly used measure of GFR nowadays. (Normal male 125 ml min⁻¹, female 110 ml min⁻¹). A 24-hour urine collection accompanied with a venous blood specimen taken (ideally) during the collection period should be sent to the laboratory.

GFR is calculated from the equation UV/P.

3 Cr⁵¹ EDTA clearance is performed by the Nuclear Medicine Department and involves an injection of labelled EDTA followed by blood samples taken at intervals to measure the rate of disappearance from the blood.

4 I¹³¹ Sodium diatrizoate clearances are measured in similar fashion in some departments.

BLOOD UREA

In assessing renal function this is one of the first tests asked for. It will not give an accurate assessment of glomerular function as it can be influenced by many exogenous factors, e.g. food intake, states of hydration, intestinal bleeding, drugs and liver function (Fig. 4.1).

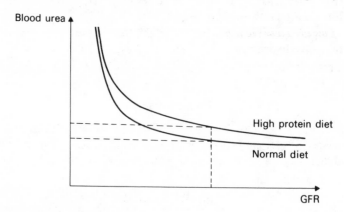

Fig. 4.1 Relationship between blood urea and GFR.

CREATININE

This gives a better indication of renal function, as it is not influenced by as many factors. Plasma creatinine levels are proportional to muscle mass, so provided body weight remains stable it gives a reasonable indication of changes in GFR.

Reciprocal of plasma creatinine (1/Cr)

An even better index of sequential renal function can be obtained by measuring the reciprocal of the plasma creatinine.

VARIATIONS IN UREA AND CREATININE

1 *High Urea, relative to creatinine*
   (a) Dehydration
   (b) Fever, infection and trauma
   (c) Drugs—corticosteroids, tetracyclines
   (d) Heart failure (diuretics)
   (e) Very high protein diet
2 *Low urea in relation to creatinine*
   (a) Low protein diet
   (b) Liver failure
   (c) Dialysis
3 *Low urea and creatinine*
   (a) Overhydration

TESTS OF TUBULAR FUNCTION

Reasons

In suspected cases of DI, nephrogenic DI, compulsive water drinking and distal tubular dysfunction as in early pyelonephritis.

Ability to concentrate

1 Fluid deprivation for 24 hours or until patient has lost 4% of body weight. Then measure urinary osmolality (normal people should concentrate to above 900 mosmol kg^{-1}).

2   Give injection of vasopressin (Pitressin or DDAVP) and measure urinary osmolality over the next eight hours. (Normal people should concentrate to above 750 mosmol kg^{-1}).

3   A useful screening test can be performed by withholding fluid overnight and testing the osmolality of the first morning specimen. A result in excess of 600 mosmol kg^{-1} would be satisfactory.

Ability to acidify

Defects in the proximal tubule result in excessive loss of bicarbonate. This loss continues until acidosis develops, when urine pH falls.

Distal tubular defects interfere with the ability to excrete titratable acid and ammonia. These patients fail to acidify urine despite severe metabolic acidosis.

Acidification test (Wrong & Davies 1959)

0.1 g ammonium chloride kg^{-1} body weight is given with 0.5 l of fluid. Plasma bicarbonate and urinary pH are then measured over the next eight hours. Normally the pH should fall below 5.3 ($H^+ > 482$ nmol/l).

Urinary bicarbonate may also be measured.

RADIOLOGY

1   Plain abdominal films and tomography often provide useful information regarding renal size and shape, the presence of radio-opaque calculi and skeletal deformities such as spina bifida which may be associated with neurological defects interfering with normal bladder function.

2   The intravenous urogram (IVU) using an iodine based contrast medium, e.g. Conray or urograffin is the standard method of outlining the shape and size of the kidneys as well as the anatomy of the collecting systems.

The quality of the images seen will depend considerably on the adequacy of renal function but with high dose infusion of contrast with tomography, surprisingly good nephrographic views can be obtained, even when renal function is very poor. No patient with impaired renal function or suspected myelomatosis should be dehydrated prior to IVU and care should be taken in diabetics for renal failure may be precipitated.

Abnormalities

(a)   In acute renal failure due to acute tubular necrosis (ATN) a prompt nephrogram will be seen which gradually fades over several hours without producing a worthwhile pyelogram.

(b)   In acute obstruction, a slowly developing nephrogram occurs, often with a negative outline of dilated calyces and pelvis. Delayed films taken 12 or 24 hours later will show retention of contrast medium in the dilated collecting system.

(c)   In chronic renal failure, the renal outlines will be poorly defined due to poor concentration in the renal tissue, but small, smooth (in glomerulonephritis) or scarred (in pyelonephritis) outlines can usually be demonstrated.

(d)   In various forms of cystic disease, compression of the cortical tissues can be shown surrounding the cysts.

(e)   In the case of tumours, bulges on the surface of the kidney or distortion of the pelvicalyceal system may be seen.

(f)   In acute glomerulonephritis a slowly developing nephrogram may be seen. No significant pyelogram develops.

ULTRASOUND

This is a technique which is very useful to assess renal position, shape and size. Cystic and solid lesions within the kidney can often be distinguished and provide a guide to their position if attempts at aspiration or biopsy are contemplated.

CT SCANNING

Further sophistication of renal imaging is offered by the CT scanner.

Micturating cystourethrography

The purpose of this investigation is to assess:
1   the size and shape of the bladder;

2 the bladder's performance during voiding;
3 the state of the bladder neck and urethra during voiding;
4 whether or not vesicoureteric reflux is occurring either during filling of the bladder or on voiding.

RENAL BIOPSY

PERCUTANEOUS RENAL BIOPSY

Introduced in 1951 by Iversen and Brun.
Indications: to determine diagnosis and decide prognosis and treatment:
1 diffuse renal disease of indeterminate aetiology, asymptomatic proteinuria or haematuria;
2 occasionally in acute renal failure where cause is unknown;
3 renal transplantation—to diagnose rejection and monitor progress.

Precautions

Check clotting factors and platelet count.
Check that two kidneys are present and functioning.
Control blood pressure.
Crossmatch two pints of blood.

Contraindications

1 Bleeding tendency, i.e. prolonged prothrombin time or platelet count $< 100\,000\,cm^{-1}m$.
2 Single functioning kidney (except in transplant cases).
3 Uncontrolled hypertension.
4 Endstage fibrotic kidneys.

Technique

Can be done blindly or under radiographic control.
X-ray of kidneys necessary to establish their position.
Lie patient prone with small pillow under abdomen.
Shoulders should be flat on the bed.

X-ray landmarks

Spinous processes.
Tip of 11th or 12th ribs.
Drop perpendicular from tip of ribs to spine and note distance of midpoint of lower pole from spine.

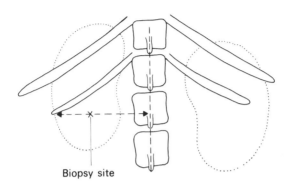

Biopsy site

Mark spot corresponding to midpoint of lower pole on back and after cleansing and draping inject local anaesthetic down to level of renal capsule. The biopsy needle (Trucut, Travenol) is introduced through the anaesthetic area down to the renal capsule. As soon as the kidney is entered, respiratory movements will cause the handle of the biopsy needle to move in a cephalad direction. The biopsy should then be taken when the patient holds his breath. The patient should then remain in bed for 24 hours under observation.

Processing of the biopsy should be undertaken immediately, portions of tissue being placed in appropriate fixatives for light microscopy, electron microscopy and immunofluorescence.

Complications

Bleeding is the most important and this occurs to a small extent in all cases. Serious haemorrhage requiring blood transfusion and/or surgical intervention is, fortunately, rare if the above mentioned pre-biopsy precautions are observed.

Chapter 5
Isotope Studies

The enthusiasm with which these are employed varies from one hospital to another and depends on the convictions of the doctors involved as well as on the availability of equipment and isotopes.

CHROMIUM Cr^{51} EDTA CLEARANCE

This is an isotopic method of assessing glomerular filtration rate. A bolus injection of Chromium^{51} EDTA is made and plasma radio-activity is measured from samples taken two, three and four hours after the initial injection. The method is more accurate than creatinine clearance when GFR is low and obviates the need for a 24-hour urine collection with its attendant inaccuracies and may be repeated serially without dangers resulting from radiation.

RENOGRAPHY

This technique uses the fact that hippuric acid is totally cleared from the blood stream by the kidney. A bolus injection of orthoiodohippuric acid is made and disappearance from the blood stream is measured by a probe placed over the chest. Uptake by the kidneys is measured by two other probes situated over the organs. Alternatively renal uptake may be measured using a gamma-camera and in this situation blood clearance is assessed by a background count around the kidneys. Since hippuran is totally cleared by the kidneys it provides an index of total renal blood flow. By measuring uptake over the two kidneys simultaneously an assessment may be made of the relative blood flow through each kidney, and the relative rates at which isotope is cleared by the kidneys. The technique has several clinical applications.

1   It provides a method of assessing the relative function of kidneys which may have suffered as a result of infection, stones, etc. Since

the radiation dose is extremely low, serial measurements may be made safely.

2   A renogram may also be used to assess obstruction by tumours fibrosis, etc. The dose of radiation is very much lower than that necessary for urography.

3   Renography is at least as sensitive and perhaps more so than IVU in detecting renal artery stenosis.

DIETHYLENETRIAMINE PENTA-ACETIC ACID (DTPA) SCAN

This technetium-labelled substance is not totally cleared and its excretion by the kidneys depends on the glomerular filtration rate. It therefore gives a nuclear equivalent of the intravenous urogram. Because relatively more counts per unit time are emitted the technique enables more information to be gleaned than from the renogram as follows:

(a)   Imaging of the arrival of the tracer into the kidney may be measured and this will give an index of whether the kidneys are perfused.

This information is useful in a patient involved in an accident where there is doubt as to renal vascularization.

(b)   Again, because of the higher count rate, the pelvicalyceal system is outlined and it is possible to see evidence of obstruction. Similarly, because the isotope can also be detected in the bladder an isotopic micturating picture may be obtained to assess whether reflux occurs.

(c)   A DTPA scan may also give an indication of acute tubular necrosis since the behaviour of the isotope is similar to the contrast medium when an intravenous urogram is performed. There is rapid renal uptake of tracer but the isotope does not get into the pelvicalyceal system but rather diffuses back into the circulation so that after about 20 minutes or so there is loss of activity.

(d)   A DTPA scan may be used to measure GFR but this requires multiple blood samples. However, since the signal to background ratio is much higher than with a renogram the accuracy of this measurement is less.

(e)   A DTPA scan is useful in the assessment of decreased renal function or anuria in patients who have undergone renal transplantation since it will often allow the differentiation between ischaemia, acute tubular necrosis and outflow obstruction.

DIMERCAPTOSUCCINIC ACID (DMSA) SCAN

This compound is selectively and slowly taken up by the renal parenchyma so that it is an ideal compound to demonstrate filling defects within the renal substance such as those produced by renal tumours or cysts. It can detect lesions greater than 1 cm in diameter. The technique is also useful where a diagnosis of renal arterial embolus is suspected since the scan will show filling defects before atrophy of the ischaemic tissue has taken place.

Chapter 6
Water and Electrolyte Balance

In health the balance of body fluids is maintained by the kidneys. The oral intake of fluids along with water produced from the metabolism of food (200–300 ml day^{-1}) is balanced by fluid losses via the skin, lungs and kidneys with a small, usually insignificant loss through the gut.

Fluid intake is governed normally by thirst. This is stimulated through the hypothalamus by the plasma osmolality and blood volume. Fluid losses via the skin and lungs are dependent upon environmental temperature, humidity, exercise, etc. The kidneys, on the other hand, are capable of adjusting output of water and salts by their own regulatory systems.

Approximate composition of tissue compartments for a 60 kg man

Total body water	60%		
Solids	40%		
Intracellular fluid (ICF)	43%		
Extracellular fluid (ECF)	17%	Interstitial 12.5%	Plasma 4.5%

(See Table 6.1).

Table 6.1 Main ionic components of ECF + ICF.

ECF	mmol l^{-1}	ICF	mmol l^{-1}
Na	135	K	164
K	4	Na	10
		Mg	28
Cl	100	PO$_4$	105
CO$_2$	27	SO$_4$	20

'Third space' fluids are those found in pleural, peritoneal cavities and the gut. Newborn babies and infants have a relatively higher proportion (65–75%) of body water than adults.

The ionic differences across cell membranes are maintained by energy pumps, e.g. the chloride pump that keeps chloride and sodium out of the cell. During periods of hypoxia and metabolic inbalance these energy sources are impaired, with the result that the pump fails and sodium accumulates inside cells whilst K^+ ions escape into the extracellular fluid. Total body fluid depends on the total ionic concentration, i.e. extracellular sodium and intracellular potassium, and as cell membranes are freely permeable to water, the amount of water in each compartment will depend, therefore, on the relative solute concentrations.

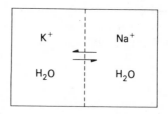

Loss or gain of Na and H_2O have more profound effects on ECF than loss or gain of H_2O alone.

Renal control of ECF concentration

The kidneys control the extracellular concentration by adjusting the excretion of sodium and of water. The capacity of the kidneys to cope with large fluctuations in sodium and water load are enormous.

When the subject is given a large intake of sodium either by mouth or intravenously, a rapid adjustment of urinary sodium excretion occurs which is independent of GFR, aldosterone excretion or ADH. This rapid adjustment is thought to be mediated by a ·naturetic hormone and it is possible that the majority of its action is on the proximal renal tubules. Where sodium intake is low, circulatory volume will be reduced and aldosterone production increased. The net result of this is to increase distal tubular sodium reabsorption until sodium balance is restored. If further increase in sodium intake occurs, the aldosterone mechanism will be reversed and diminished reabsorption will occur at the distal tubule and concomitantly there will be a diminution in the production of renin by the kidney. Hormones such as parathyroid hormone and calcitonin (which both increase cyclic AMP production by the proximal tubular cells) can inhibit net sodium reabsorption but they probably play a very small part in normal sodium homeostasis.

Control of water is closely linked with that of sodium. Normal subjects require approximately 800 ml of fluid per day to remain in water balance. If they drink less, they tend to become dehydrated, and if uncorrected this will lead to a diminished glomerular filtration rate and retention of metabolic waste products. If the volume of water ingested is increased, plasma osmolality falls, thus inhibiting antidiuretic hormone release and making the distal collecting duct impervious to water with large volumes of dilute urine to be passed each day. States of dehydration, conversely, will stimulate ADH release and increase collecting duct permeability resulting in reabsorption of water by the distal tubules.

Clinical assessment of patients with suspected water and electrolyte disturbances

1   Clinical history including drug intake, operations, vomiting, diarrhoea.

2   Clinical examination with particular regard to the following:
  (a) state of peripheral perfusion—temperature, cyanosis, sweatiness;
  (b) lying and standing blood pressure and character of pulse;
  (c) state of tongue, tissue turgor and eyeball tension;
  (d) jugular venous pressure (JVP) (or central venous pressure (CVP));
  (e) presence or absence of oedema;
  (f) level of consciousness;
  (g) abnormal sites of fluid loss;
  (h) chart intake and output as well as daily weight.

3   Biochemical assessment:
  (a) blood urea, electrolytes, creatinine;
  (b) urinary electrolytes, urea, protein;
  (c) haematocrit (packed cell volume (PCV));

  (d) plasma H^+ ion concentration, P_aO_2, P_aCO_2;

  (e) simultaneous plasma and urine osmolalities.

4   Bacteriology.

  (a) culture of blood;

  (b) midstream urine (MSU);

  (c) wounds;

  (d) sputum;

  (e) stools (if appropriate).

5   ECG, chest X-ray.

A normal healthy individual during the course of 24 hours would drink daily 1.5 litres of fluid; his food would contribute 300 ml of water of metabolism, making his total intake 1.8 litres. Insensible losses, i.e. via skin, lungs and gut, would be 400 ml in a temperate climate and urine output would be expected to be about 1.4 litres, thus maintaining fluid balance.

In many clinical situations this balance can be upset. Healthy kidneys will adjust urine output in a variety of environmental situations but as impairment of renal function occurs this facility may be lost and environmental factors take on a more important role (Table 6.2).

Table 6.2   Clinical assessment of patients' fluid balance.

Clinical situations	Consequence
fever and sweating	water loss predominantly
vomiting, nasogastric (NG) aspiration	water H^+ Na^+ K^+ Cl' losses
intestinal fistulae	water Na^+ K^+ HCO_3' losses
diarrhoea	water Na^+ and K^+ lost
hyperventilation	water and H^+ lost
chronic renal failure	(water) Na^+ K^+ lost sometimes
acute $\}$ renal failure chronic	water Na^+ and K^+ retention
hypoxia	H^+ retention
underventilation	H^+ retention

Remember that an increased rate of catabolism in renal failure, particularly if infection is present, will lead to excessive tissue breakdown and the release of K^+, urea and H^+ into the ECF.

The most important electrolyte disturbances are those in which salt and water are retained or lost in isotonic proportions, conditions known as overhydration (or saline excess) and dehydration (saline depletion).

Pure water excess or depletion are rare in healthy states.

Water excess

Caused by administration of excess water, usually intravenously as hypotonic saline or 5% glucose. Patients in coma, renal failure or who have just undergone surgical operations are susceptible. Inappropriate ADH secretion can occur in many conditions, e.g. after head injuries, after cerebrovascular accidents, meningitis, TB, carcinoma of the bronchus, pneumonia, hypothyroidism etc. and can lead to states of water intoxication.

Consequences

Plasma sodium concentration falls and ECF becomes hypotonic so that water shifts into cells, particularly in the brain. Drowsiness, muscle weakness, nausea, vomiting and convulsions can occur.

Treatment is by withholding water. Occasionally hypertonic sodium chloride needs to be administered slowly.

Water depletion

Caused by decreased intake or increased losses. Patients stuporose or in coma, after strokes when they cannot communicate, infants with nephrogenic DI and patients in chronic renal failure are susceptible.

Conscious patients become thirsty and hypernatraemia is found but hypotension and low tissue turgor are absent until very late.

Treatment consists of administering 5% glucose with care.

Saline excess

Causes—excessive intake of sodium
inability to excrete sodium

Excess intake of sodium occurs very rarely. It is occasionally seen in infants and in unconscious patients fed compounds with inappropriately high sodium concentrations. Inadvertently hypertonic saline may be infused or a dialysis patient may be dialysed against too high a sodium concentration.

Clinical signs—irritability, hypertonia, hypertension, coma.

Treatment

1 Glucose or mannitol infusions containing potassium.
2 Dialysis.

Oedema

The appearance of oedema indicates at least overloading to the tune of the equivalent of 3 litres of normal saline. Sodium retention leading to oedema is usually found in:

(a) renal failure;
(b) nephrotic syndrome;
(c) hepatic failure;
(d) cardiac failure;
(e) pregnancy;
(f) Drugs, e.g. carbenoxolone, methyl dopa, etc.

It can be the result of (a) diminished GFR as in renal failure; (b) secondary hyperaldosteronism.

The presence of oedema despite a low plasma sodium always indicates saline excess.

Treatment

1 Reduce sodium intake.
2 Promote sodium and water losses by diuretics.
3 Use aldosterone antagonist, e.g. spironolactone.
4 Restore plasma volume by protein infusion if appropriate.
5 Use drugs to improve cardiac output.
6 Drain pleural effusions, ascites, etc.
7 Stop offending drugs.

Saline depletion

Renal causes—tubular disorders:

1 renal failure
2 pyelonephritis
3 polycystic disease
4 interstitial nephritis
5 chronic urinary tract
   obstruction (when relieved)

Extrarenal causes:

1 diarrhoea, e.g. cholera, intestinal fistulae
2 excessive diuretic use
3 osmotic diuresis e.g. diabetes mellitus
4 Addison's disease
5 fibrocystic disease
6 ? loss by sweat
7 dialysis

Patients with impaired renal function are particularly susceptible to sodium losses.

Symptoms

Lethargy, cramps, loss of appetite, muscle weakness, postural hypotension.

Signs

Low tissue turgor and eyeball pressure, dry tongue, low JVP and postural hypotension.
PCV will rise.

Treatment

1 Replace deficit with saline initially. Transfuse until JVP (or CVP) and blood pressure (BP) are satisfactory (usually at least 3 L deficient).
2 Monitor body weight and renal function frequently. Long-term treatment includes assessment of patient's urinary capacity to excrete sodium and arrange intake accordingly. This may fluctuate considerably. Use Na Cl (17 mmol g^{-1}), Na bicarbonate (12 mmol g^{-1}) or slow Na (10 mmol).
Combined saline and water depletion is seen at its worst in hyperosmolar ketotic diabetes. The intense glucose diuresis is responsible. Saline depletion and hypernatraemia occur.

Potassium

K^+ is the most important intracellular cation, 98% of total body K^+ being within cells. 3.5–5 mmol l^{-1} remain in the extracellular compartment and fluctuations outside these limits may have profound effects on neuromuscular and cardiac function.

Hyperkalaemia (elevated plasma potassium)

Causes

(a) Diminished renal excretion as in renal failure (GFR < 10 ml min^{-1}). Clinically more important in acute than chronic renal failure.
(b)   Shift of intracellular → extracellular K^+ as in metabolic acidosis, during muscular exertion and in catabolic states, e.g. burns, septicaemia;
(c)   Due to excessive intake of K^+ containing foods, medicines and K^+-conserving diuretics, also i/v K^+ and blood transfusion;
(d)   In Addisons disease;
   The main clinical effect is on heart muscle and this can only be determined by ECG monitoring. The first event may be cardiac arrest. ECG changes include those shown in Fig. 6.1. Weakness and sometimes paralysis of skeletal muscle can occur.

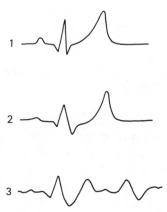

Fig. 6.1   ECG in hyperkalaemia.

Other ECG changes are:
1 symmetrical peaked T waves;
2 widening of QRS complexes and flattening of P waves;
3 ventricular fibrillation.

Treatment

1 Protect the myocardium with 1–2 g calcium gluconate or chloride intravenously;
2 Encourage K^+ to return to the cells
  (a) 50 g glucose and 20 units soluble insulin, both i/v;
  (b) intravenous sodium bicarbonate (take care not to overload with sodium in cases of renal failure);
3 Dialyse;

MAINTENANCE

1 Exchange resins, e.g. calcium resonium 15 g tds. (Orally or rectally. A laxative such as lactulose should be given to prevent constipation.);
2 Potassium-losing diuretics, e.g. frusemide;
3 Low K^+ diet;
4 Avoid K^+ containing drugs and K^+ conserving diuretics.

Hypokalaemia

Potassium depletion occurs as a result of:
1 decreased potassium intake.
2 increased renal losses
  (a) renal tubular acidosis and Fanconi syndrome;
  (b) metabolic alkalosis;
  (c) primary and secondary aldosteronism;
  (d) corticosteroid therapy;
  (e) diuretic therapy with inadequate K^+ replacement;
  (f) in osmotic diuresis, e.g. uncontrolled diabetes mellitus.
3 Gastro-intestinal (GI) losses, e.g. diarrhoea, excessive laxative intake, intestinal fistulae and K^+ secreting tumours.

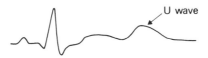

Fig. 6.2   ECG in hypokalaemia.

Symptoms due to hypokalaemia occur when serum K^+ $<2.5\,\mathrm{mmol}\,1^{-1}$, and include muscular weakness and fatigue. Muscles are hypotonic and reflexes are depressed. Flaccid paralysis occurs in extreme cases. ECG shows flattened T waves and the appearance of U waves (Fig. 6.2). ST depression and QRS widening also occurs. Cardiac muscle becomes more susceptible to the action of cardiac glycosides, e.g. digitalis. Abdominal distension, constipation and paralytic ileus may be present. Respiratory failure can occur.

Hypokalaemia produces distal renal tubular abnormalities with cellular vacuolation and loss of concentrating ability.

Assessment of K^+ depletion can be difficult for plasma K^+ levels may not always be depressed. Careful measurement of urinary and intestinal losses are important. Remember that in severe K^+ depletion, H^+ will be excreted by the renal tubular cells thus making the urine acid and leading to extracellular alkalosis. When the kidneys are the source of K^+ loss, H^+ will be retained and the urine will be neutral or alkaline.

Treatment

In states of depletion $300–1000\,\mathrm{mmol}\,K^+$ need to be replaced.
1   If diuretics are responsible, add K^+ conserving agents, e.g. spironolactone or amiloride.
2   Oral K^+ replacement—slow K (8 mmol K^+/tabs), effervescent K^+ (6.5 mmol/tab) or Kloref (6.7 mmol/tabs), Sando-K (12 mmol/tabs). Be sure to give enough.
3   It may be necessary to give K^+ intravenously. This should be diluted with saline or glucose to a maximum concentration $30–40\,\mathrm{mmol}\,1^{-1}$. This should be infused slowly over 2–3 h.
Maximum daily dose $150–250\,\mathrm{mmol}\,\mathrm{day}^{-1}$.
In the presence of renal impairment these doses should be reduced.

Acid-base balance

Dietary protein metabolism leads to the production of $70\,\mathrm{mmol}\,H^+$ day^{-1} (non-volatile acids—SO_4 and PO_4). Most organic acids are metabolized to CO_2 and H_2O. CO_2 is excreted via the lungs, non-metabolized acids, organic and inorganic, are dissociated in body fluids, the ionic components being excreted by the kidneys. The H^+

ions are excreted exclusively by the tubules. The concentration of H^+ in the body determines acid-base status.

Acid	Source
H_2CO_3	CHO, fat and protein
H_2SO_4 ⎱ H_3PO_4 ⎰	protein, phospholipids
keto ⎱ lactic ⎰ acids oxalic ⎰	protein, and incomplete oxidation of fat and carbohydrate

Sulphur content of the diet contributes to majority of non-volatile H^+ production and in tissue hypoxia and diabetes mellitus, lactic acid and keto acids are produced in increased quantities thus putting an extra load on the kidneys.

Buffer systems

The acid produced at the site of metabolism is buffered before being transported to the kidney for excretion. Intracellularly, proteins act as buffers whereas bicarbonate acts as the main extracellular buffer. Inside red cells reduced haemoglobin acts as a buffer. Bicarbonate allows for rapid removal of H^+ by the lungs and also transports H^+ into the red cells for buffering by haemoglobin. Other plasma buffers such as phosphate are only called into play when the primary buffers are saturated.

Excretion of hydrogen ions

This occurs both in the proximal and distal renal tubules. H^+ is derived from H_2CO_3 produced in tubular cells by the hydration of CO_2 under the influence of carbonic anhydrase. In the proximal tubules, H^+ is excreted in combination with bicarbonate filtered by the glomeruli ($5000 \, mmol \, day^{-1}$). In the distal tubules H^+ is excreted as titratable acid bound to phosphate (HPO_4^{11} and $H_2PO_4^{1}$), and bound to ammonia, NH_3 being derived from the deamination of glutamine in the distal tubular cells.

Normally approximately 30 mmol of titratable acid and 40 mmol of NH_{4+} are excreted daily but the kidney is capable of increasing NH_4^+ excretion to over 200 mmols if necessary. Therefore total acid output is a combination of titratable acid, and ammonium minus unneutralized bicarbonate that might appear in the urine.

Acidosis

Acidosis can occur as a result of selective renal tubular defects which are classified as Types I and II depending upon whether the functional abnormality is in the distal or proximal tubule respectively.

In Type I renal tubular acidosis, (RTA), the distal tubule fails to maintain the normal H^+ gradient between urine and plasma, so that tubular acidosis is reduced and the urine contains bicarbonate. Hypokalaemia is common. Impairment of renal function is unusual but urinary tract infection and nephrocalcinosis may occur. Prognosis is usually good but failure to acidify and concentrate urine often leads to problems of fluid and electrolyte balance as well as renal stone formation and osteomalacia. It may be inherited as a Mendelian Dominant or be acquired as a result of tubular damage due to obstruction, hypercalcaemia or urinary infections. Treatment by alkalis and K^+ supplements will prevent or cure the osteomalacia or rickets. Potassium citrate mixtures are suitable. Surgical treatment of renal stones may be necessary and orthopaedic treatment for fractures.

Type II RTA is due to a disordered function of the proximal tubular cells. These cells are unable to excrete hydrogen ions so that most of the filtered bicarbonate appears in the urine. Urine pH is high and hypokalaemia and osteomalacia may occur. Treatment with alkalis is usually disappointing. This condition occurs more commonly in infants than in adults. In the former it appears to be an isolated defect and sometimes transient. In adults other tubular abnormalities may accompany it, e.g. Fanconi's syndrome, Wilson's disease, cystinosis, hyperparathyroidism and intoxication with degraded tetracyclines.

Uraemic acidosis

In advanced renal failure H^+ cannot be adequately excreted due to the inability of the tubular cells of the kidneys to excrete phosphate and to produce ammonia. Treatment with Na bicarbonate can be dangerous

(a) because of the risk of sodium overloading;

(b) because of the risk of tetany.

Chapter 7
Acute Renal Failure

This is usually recognized by a sudden reduction in urinary output to below 400 ml per day, accompanied by the accumulation of metabolic waste products in the blood.

Causes

In clinical practice acute renal failure may be seen in many circumstances. By far the most common antecedent events are related to traumatic injuries, blood loss, surgical operation, septicaemias and drugs or poisons. Rarely, certain acute forms of glomerulonephritis, malignant hypertension, acute pyelonephritis and haemolytic uraemic syndrome can lead to acute renal failure. Obstruction to the lower urinary tract should always be excluded (Table 7.1).

Table 7.1 Causes of acute renal failure.

Vascular	Parenchymal	Obstruction
Renal arterial occlusion: (a) thrombosis, (b) embolus	Glomerulitis	Stones
	Necrotizing arteritis: (a) Polyarteritis nodosa (PAN) (b) Henoch-Schönlein purpura (HSP)	Casts
Renal vein thrombosis		Crystals
	Haemolytic uraemic syndrome	Pelvi-ureteric junction (PUJ) obstruction
	Malignant hypertension, scleroderma	Bladder neck obstruction
	Acute pyelonephritis	Tumours
	Transplant rejection	Fibrosis
	Acute tubular necrosis, (ATN)	TB and schistosomiasis

Most cases of acute renal failure follow some vascular accident resulting in circulatory insufficiency, e.g. cardiogenic, hypovolaemic or septicaemic shock. Drugs and poisons are sometimes responsible. This form of renal failure is called 'acute tubular necrosis' (ATN) or vasomotor nephropathy. Early awareness of impending trouble, e.g. bleeding, and its prompt treatment with blood transfusion to restore blood volume will often prevent renal failure. The degree of circulatory disturbance and its duration are both important from the point of view of developing renal damage.

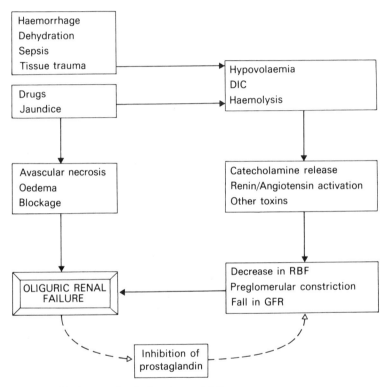

Fig. 7.1 Pathogenesis of oliguric renal failure.

Pathophysiology of ATN

1 Tubular changes

Tubular cell damage has been recognized for years in ischaemic and nephrotoxic renal failure, the former showing patchy cell destruction including the basement membrane, the latter more generalized cellular damage but leaving the basement membrane intact. However, in many cases of renal failure no definitive tubular damage can be recognized.

2 Back diffusion

Back diffusion of tubular fluid via damaged tubular cells into interstitium probably occurs and contributes to interstitial oedema seen histologically.

3 Tubular blockage

Tubular blockage by cell debris and proteins is important in renal failure due to myelomatosis and nephrotoxins.

4 Renal vasoconstriction

This is probably the most important contributing factor in ATN. Trueta (1947) showed that stimulation of the sympathetic nerves to the kidneys of rabbits caused cortical vasoconstriction similar to that which occurred in hypotension and trauma. Radioisotope and micropuncture techniques have confirmed cortical ischaemia with medullary shunting. The renal blood flow in this situation is 30–40% of normal whereas GFR is less than $5\,\mathrm{ml\,min^{-1}}$.

5 Disseminated intravascular coagulation

This undoubtedly occurs in patients with extensive tissue damage and sepsis. The release of cellular and bacterial toxins (endotoxin) into the circulation triggers off the coagulation cascade and initiates the release of vasoactive substances.

6 Prostaglandins

Prostaglandins normally produced by the renal medulla probably play an important regulatory role in controlling afferent arteriolar tone. When urine flow is stopped their transport to the cortex ceases and uninhibited arteriolar vasoconstriction will occur.

Clinical course

Five stages of ATN have been described:

1 Onset

During this period the patient presents often with multisystem problems, e.g. extensive trauma, sepsis, haemorrhage, pulmonary and central nervous system (CNS) damage, etc. All efforts are made to resuscitate the patient and *en passant* it might be noticed that urine output is adequate or that plasma urea and creatinine are rising.

Prompt action to restore blood volume or to correct electrolyte disturbances might result in rapid recovery of normal renal function. If not the patient enters the next phase.

2 Oliguric or anuric phase

Urine output remains at 400 ml day^{-1} or less. During this period metabolic waste products, salt and water accumulate in the blood, so that dialysis treatment is usually necessary. This phase may last for up to 6 weeks.

3 Early diuretic phase

Here urine output begins to increase and there is a slow improvement in GFR. This phase continues until the blood urea begins spontaneously to fall and dialysis is usually necessary throughout.

4 Late diuretic phase

This is the phase during which blood urea concentrations fall to their ultimate level. Dialysis treatment is, therefore, gradually withdrawn and special care of fluid and electrolyte balance is important. Though the GFR may recover well during this phase, renal tubular function remains poor and may take months or years to reach optimum levels.

5 Convalescent phase

This lasts several months during which time the patient returns to his normal self.

Metabolic consequences of renal failure

1 Water and salt imbalance

A common complication is overhydration leading to peripheral oedema and pulmonary oedema. This is due to inappropriate salt and water intake. Strict attention should be paid to intake and output charts and the patients should be weighed daily. In nonoliguric renal failure or where there are large gastrointestinal losses, dehydration may become a problem.

2 Hyperkalaemia

This is a dangerous consequence of renal failure for it can lead to cardiac arrhythmias. It is likely to be a problem in patients suffering from widespread tissue damage (traumatic or ischaemic) and where the rate of catabolism is very high, as for example in patients with septicaemia. Severe acidosis is usually accompanied by hyperkalaemia.

3 Hypocalcaemia

This is common and is often related to a low plasma albumin. It is probably partly due to phosphate retention.

4 Metabolic acidosis

This is caused by the inability of the kidneys to excrete hydrions as well as by their excess production by the catabolism of endogenous protein and anaerobic metabolism of ischaemic tissue. It is often accompanied by hyperkalaemia.

5 Retention of breakdown products of protein metabolism

In the absence of significant renal function the products of protein breakdown accumulate in the body and are reflected by a rise in the blood levels of urea, creatinine, uric acid, guanidinosuccinic acids, phenols, enols and amines. Not only are they markers of renal decompensation but they probably contribute to many of the symptoms of renal failure, e.g. gastrointestinal disorders and bleeding tendency.

6   Haematology

A normocytic normochromic anaemia and leucocytosis are common. Renal failure inhibits erythropoiesis and also diminshes erythrocyte survival time. Platelet counts are normal unless disseminated intravascular coagulation (DIC) is present but platelet adhesiveness is abnormally low.

Clinical features

The causes of ATN themselves often pose formidable management problems, e.g. multiple bony fractures, muscle damage, major vascular disruption, pulmonary and CNS damage. In addition one has to cope with specific symptoms related to the renal failure.

(*a*) *Cardiorespiratory.*   Dyspnoea due to heart failure and arrythmias due to potassium intoxication. Pericarditis occurs rarely and may give praecordial pain. Acidosis produces the typical Kussmaul respiration (air hunger).

(*b*) *Gastrointestinal.*   Hiccoughs, anorexia, nausea, vomiting or diarrhoea occur fairly frequently.

(*c*) *Neurological.*   Headaches, stupor, agitation, drowsiness and confusion relate to the height of the plasma urea and creatinine. If untreated, myoclonic twitching and convulsions will occur and the patient lapses into coma and dies.

(*d*) *Metabolic.*   As a result of gastrointestinal disturbances and hypercatabolism, malnutrition is a very common accompaniment of severe prolonged ATN.

Management

Initial assessment

History and examination may give clues regarding aetiology. Past and family history may point to previous renal abnormalities and drug history if essential. Examination will reveal:

(a)   evidence of trauma, shock or surgical operations;

(b)   congenital defects which may be associated with renal abnormalities;

(c)   evidence suggestive of chronic renal failure, e.g. skin pigmentation, anaemia, pericarditis or peripheral neuropathy;

(d)   suggestive evidence of urinary obstruction.

Incipient renal failure

Two conditions that may easily be reversible are:
(a) hypovolaemic shock, and
(b) bladder neck or urethral obstruction.

Lower urinary obstruction can be tolerated for an amazingly long time but unless 'shock' due to hypovolaemia or any other cause is treated promptly (certainly within 12 hours) renal failure may become established. The presence of postural hypotension and a low central venous or left atrial (pulmonary wedge) pressure should be signals for urgent treatment with plasma expanders with or without mannitol or loop diuretics. Comparison of urine and plasma osmolality and urea along with urinary sodium excretion (Table 7.2) will help in determining whether renal failure is established or not.

Table 7.2   To distinguish between incipient and established renal failure.

	Incipient	Established
U_{os}/P_{os}	> 1.1	< 1.1
Urine Na^+ (mmol d^{-1})	< 20	> 40
U_{urea}/P_{urea}	$> 10:1$	$< 10:1$
FE_{Na}*	< 1	> 3

* FE_{Na} (fractional excretion of sodium).

$$= \frac{P_{Cr} \times U_{Na}}{P_{Na} \times U_{Cr}} \times 100$$

P_{Cr} = plasma creatinine (mmol l^{-1})
U_{Cr} = urinary creatinine (mmol l^{-1}).

If restoring volume results in the restoration of urine flow, fluid and diuretic therapy should be continued until normal homeostasis returns. If restoration of blood volume does not improve cardiac output and renal function, inotropic agents such as dopamine are sometimes valuable. It is interesting that dopamine is effective in promoting urine flows at infusion rates less than are required for its cardiac effect. (e.g. 2–3 μgkg^{-1}min^{-1}.)

The relief of chronic obstruction to the urinary tract may be followed by a brisk sodium diuresis and unless appropriate replacement of sodium is given the patient may become severely depleted, with resulting tubular necrosis.

ESTABLISHED RENAL FAILURE

The management of these patients can be exceedingly difficult and calls for the highest possible grade of nursing and medical care. It is therefore best conducted in an intensive care department where facilities are available for cardiac and respiratory support as well as haemodialysis and parenteral nutrition. In addition, the surgical treatment of damaged tissue, internal bleeding and drainage of abscesses may well be necessary.

Fluid and electrolyte balance

In the oliguric renal failure patients, overhydration is a major hazard and frequently patients present to a renal department already in this stage. Fluid loss in an average sized person living in a temperate climate amounts to 400–500 ml per day so that the basic allowance for such a patient should be no more than 400 ml added to the measured fluid losses for the previous day. In calculating fluid losses it is important not to ignore gastrointestinal losses such as vomiting, drainage from peritoneal and fistula sites and diarrhoea. It should be remembered that endogenous protein catabolism contributes 200–300 ml of water daily and if the patient is able to take solid food, a significant amount of water of metabolism is produced likewise.

In addition to water retention, sodium retention occurs in these patients with resulting oedema, heart failure and hypertension. Sodium allowances should, therefore, be kept to a bare minimum. This usually means 20–30 mmol per day. The finding of hyponatraemia in a patient with fluid overload never represents sodium deficiency. On the contrary, this is a dilutional hyponatraemia in a patient who is already overburdened with sodium. To give more sodium to correct the hyponatraemia would be exceedingly dangerous. The right treatment in that situation is to restrict fluid intake.

In patients with excessive vomiting, the loss of chloride and hydrogen ions can be excessive and care should be taken to replace chloride under those circumstances.

The retention of potassium and high blood levels are common in acute renal failure. Not only are the kidneys unable to excrete potassium, but as a result of tissue damage, infection and haemorrhage, endogenous potassium release from intracellular sources can cause very rapid and fatal rises in the blood level. If untreated, this can lead to cardiac arrhythmias and asystole. Treatment of such a situation is an emergency (see p. 44). If the patient remains hypercatabolic, dialysis may be the only way of effectively controlling serum potassium.

Metabolic acidosis

This is a condition that does not as a rule require active treatment. The patient may exhibit air hunger but is not particularly distressed by it. Doctors often treat this with sodium bicarbonate but the danger of sodium overloading far outweighs the danger of acidosis to the patient. In addition tetany may be precipitated if there is hypocalcaemia. As acidosis is often an accompaniment of hyperkalaemia, dialysis is the best way of controlling this.

Nutrition

Hypercatabolic patients in renal failure very rapidly become wasted, and as a result of this negative nitrogen balance, they become susceptible to infection and their state of mobility is greatly impaired.

Though the need for high calorific intake is appreciated, the practical difficulty of administering it can provide a major challenge. In the absence of available dialysis facilities it is almost impossible to administer adequate calories to such a patient, who will need at least 3000–3500 kcal per day containing 60–80 g protein of high biological value. The excess fluid that has to be administered needs to be ultrafiltrated by means of an artificial kidney. If the patient can take food by mouth, so much the better, otherwise the administration of high concentration sugar solutions and intralipid through a central catheter will be essential.

Antibiotics

Infections are a major complication of acute renal failure and so great care must be taken of wounds, pressure sores and intravenous catheter sites. There is no justification for the insertion of bladder catheters which serve only to introduce infections. Frequent cultures should be taken from all these sites along with blood cultures and chest X-rays. Prophylactic broad-spectrum antibiotics should be avoided, by and large, but proven infections should be urgently and comprehensively treated with appropriate antibiotics. Intravenous drip sites should be changed frequently.

Great care should be taken in the prescription of toxic antibiotics in renal failure. The route of excretion of all potentially toxic antibiotics should be known and wherever possible doses should be monitored by blood level measurement. Furthermore, drugs that are nephrotoxic should always be avoided if possible.

Anaemia

The treatment of anaemia rarely requires transfusion unless there has been massive blood loss or haemolysis. The restoration of blood volume, however, by plasma or plasma substitute is sometimes important.

Dialysis

Survival of many patients with hypercatabolic renal failure will depend on the availability of dialysis. Where no haemodialysis facilities are available, peritoneal dialysis may well be lifesaving. But in some cases, it may be too inefficient to control the metabolic build-up of waste products. Haemodialysis if available, should be started at a fairly early stage, before blood urea and creatinine levels rise too high. The reason for this is that bleeding tendencies come into their own in patients with blood urea levels over $35\,\mathrm{mmol\,l^{-1}}$ (more than $200\,\mathrm{mg}\,\,100\,\mathrm{ml^{-1}}$). In addition, hyperkalaemia and acidosis will be easily controlled and fluid imbalance corrected. Almost daily dialysis may well be required over the first ten days or so of the patient's course.

Diuretic phase

After the period of oliguria is over, diuresis is occurring, and GFR will recover slowly. Dialysis should be continued until a definite spontaneous improvement occurs in the blood and urine biochemistry. Daily assessment of fluid and electrolyte replacement will have to be continued during this period of time, as one must remember renal tubular function may take a long time to return to normal.

Chapter 8
Renal Glomerular Disease
(Glomerulonephritis)

INTRODUCTION

Glomerulonephritis is not a single entity but a spectrum of diseases which may be limited to the kidneys, or part of a generalized disease such as disseminated lupus erythematosus (DLE) or polyarteritis. Since very little is known about the aetiology of the various forms of glomerulonephritis, we must content ourselves with classifying them into groups on the basis of

(a)   possible underlying immune mechanisms;
(b)   the renal biopsy appearances; and
(c)   the clinical syndrome,

in the hope that these might provide information about the natural history of the different types and the possible influence of various forms of treatment. Unfortunately, as we will see later, these three classifications are not mutually supportive and there is considerable overlap.

These classifications are less satisfactory than those that depend on aetiology and this is undoubtedly why most students find it difficult to even understand the subject let alone regurgitate it in examinations. The situation is analogous to that which our forefathers suffered when they wrestled with the minutiae of lung pathology in pneumonia in the days before the organisms were understood.

THE IMMUNOLOGICAL BASIS OF GLOMERULONEPHRITIS

Immune complex nephritis

This is currently thought to be the most common mechanism of renal damage in glomerulonephritis.

(a)   What is meant by immune complex nephritis? Exogenous or endogenous antigens stimulate antibody production and either soluble antigen–antibody complexes become deposited in the kidney or, alternatively, the antigen alone becomes fixed to part of the glomerulus and the antibody to it becomes complexed to it at the site of fixation.

(b)   What evidence is there to support the idea of immune complex nephritis? Electron microscopy reveals immune complex deposition and it has been possible to extract and identify the antigenic component. The immunoglobulin fraction of the antibody may be demonstrated by immunofluorescence where it shows up as granular staining in the glomerulus. Although it is possible to detect immune complexes in the circulation it does not necessarily mean that they are responsible for glomerular disease.

(c)   How do immune complexes cause renal damage? Once an immune complex is formed it may have the capacity to activate many mediator systems particularly through a portion of the immunoglobulin molecules. The complement systems (see below), the Hageman factor system and neutrophil-dependent mechanisms of tissue damage may all be involved. What is perhaps surprising is not that immune complexes may cause glomerulonephritis, but that this does not occur more frequently.

Antiglomerular basement membrane disease (Goodpasture's Syndrome)

This rare condition is characterized by pulmonary haemorrhage and renal disease. Antibodies to glomerular and pulmonary basement membrane have been demonstrated in both the serum and glomerular eluates. The initial stimulus to the antibody production is unknown but may be infective in origin and once it has occurred seems to be, at least in part, self perpetuating. Plasmapheresis provides a means of removing the antibody and interrupting this cycle. Deposition of antibody in glomerulus may be demonstrated by immunofluorescence but unlike immune complex disease, the deposition is linear rather than granular.

Other mechanisms

In minimal-change nephropathy and certain conditions where the abnormalities occur focally, the nature of the underlying immune mechanisms is not clear, for immunofluorescence studies do not show deposition of immunoglobulin or complement in glomeruli and antiglomerular antibodies cannot be detected.

THE ROLE OF THE COMPLEMENT SYSTEM IN GLOMERULAR INJURY

Complement (c) is an enzymatic system of serum proteins which is activated in sequence by many antigen–antibody reactions and which is essential for antibody-mediated immune haemolysis. It plays a part in several other biological reactions including phagocytosis, opsonization, chemotaxis and immune adherence leading to tissue damage. The system may be activated by either the classic or alternative pathways leading to the breakdown of C3, and thence by a common pathway involving factors 5 to 9.

What is the evidence for the involvement of the complement system in glomerular disease?

(a)   There is a decrease in the concentration of serum complement components.

(b)   Complement components may be demonstrated in the glomeruli.

(c)   Blood contains complement breakdown products.

(d)   Using the technique of radiolabelled C3, changes can be shown in the rate of synthesis and degradation of this in certain forms of glomerulonephritis.

Classic pathway activation of complement occurs notably in systemic lupus erythematosus (SLE) and in certain bacterial infections. The stimulus to activation seems to be the immune complexes themselves and evidence that it has occurred is adduced by low levels of C1, C2 and C4 in the blood. Alternative pathway activation occurs in Type 2 mesangiocapillary glomerulonephritis and also in IgA (Berger) disease. In the former it seems that an IgG autoantibody known as C3 nephritic factor is the initiating factor. With this type of activation the C1, 2 and 4 levels are normal in the presence of decreased levels of C3 factor B and properdin.

As well as complement being involved in glomerular damage, there is an increased incidence of renal glomerular disease in patients suffering from certain complement deficiencies:

(a)   patients with C3 deficiency may suffer from mesangiocapillary glomerular disease and, in some, C3 neph may be found in the blood;

Table 8.1 Histological changes in various forms of glomerulonephritis

	Clinical	Proteinuria	Haematuria	LM	IF	EM
Normal	Normal	nil	nil	N	N	N
Min.-change	Nephrotic	+	–	N	N	Foot process fusion
Diffuse prolif.	Acute nephritis	+	+	Prolif.	C3 IgG	Epithelial cells and sub-epithelial humps
Focal prolif.	Haematuria (proteinuria) Bergers, HSP SBE, PAN, SLE	+	+	Focal prolif.	IgA/G	unhelpful
Focal sclerosis	Nephrotic Proteinuria CRF	+	+	Hyalinosis	IgM/C_3	unhelpful
Membranous	Nephrotic CRF	+	–	BM spikes	Granular IgG/M	BM deposit
Membrano-prolif.	Shunt neph PLD	+	+	Thick BM, split + cells	Granular IgG/M	Type I split BM Type 2 dense deposits
Crescentic	Goodpasture's Polyarteritis, etc. Renal failure	+	+	Crescents	Fibrin in cres.	

N, normal; BM, basement membrane; HSP, Henoch-Schölein Purpura; SBE, subacute bacterial endocarditis; PAN, polyarteritis nodosa; SLE, systemic (or disseminated) lupus erythematosus; CRF, chronic renal failure; PLD, partial lipodystrophy.

(b) in hereditary angio-oedema, C1 esterase inhibitor deficiency occurs, and mesangiocapillary glomerulonephritis is also more commonly found in these patients.

Renal biopsy appearances

Most people find terms like membranous, mesangiocapillary or focal sclerosis confusing and difficult to remember since they have no knowledge of the pathological changes to which the terms refer. This section briefly outlines the histological changes which are seen in the various forms of glomerulonephritis (Table 8.1).

Renal tissue usually obtained by biopsy (see p. 31) is examined not only by the light microscope but also by the electron microscope and, in addition, frozen sections are stained with fluorescein-labelled antibodies against immunoglobulins, fibrin, complement components, etc.

Glossary of terms

Focal: changes which occur to a much greater extent in some glomeruli compared with others.

Segmental: changes present in one or more parts of the glomerulus while the remainder is normal or only mildly affected.

Proliferation: an increase in the number of cells. May affect only part of the glomerulus, e.g. mesangial proliferation or epithelial proliferation.

Crescents: multiple layers of cells deposited between the tuft and Bowman's capsule that encircle and encroach on the glomerular tuft. The cells are derived from the parietal epithelium.

1   Minimal-change glomerulonephritis (lipoid nephrosis)

This is the commonest cause of the nephrotic syndrome (NS) in children but is also seen in adults. Under the light microscope the kidney appears normal but electron microscopy shows fusion of foot processes. Immunofluorescent staining for immunoglobulin, complement, etc., is negative.

2   Membranous glomerulonephritis (extramembranous or epimembranous GN)

This is an example of immune complex glomerulonephritis. Where the antigen is unidentified it is known as idiopathic, but in the following conditions, the antigenic stimulus is recognized as shown in Table 8.2.

Table 8.2   Recognized antigenic stimulus.

Associated disease	Antigen
Post-streptococcal glomerulonephritis	Streptococcal antigen
Bacterial endocarditis	Infecting organisms, e.g. *Streptococcus viridans*, *Staphylococcus aureus*
Infected shunt	Infecting organism *Staphylococcus albus*
Malaria	*Plasmodium malariae*
Hepatitis	Australia Antigen B
Drugs	Penicillamine, gold, Troxidone, etc.
Carcinoma	Carcinoma antigen
DLE	DNA and RNA
Cryoglobulinaemia	Immunoglobulin

The light-microscopic appearance shows thickening of the capillary loops and these, when thin sections stained with silver are examined, appear to have a spiky appearance. On electron-microscopy sub-epithelial deposits are visible in the glomerular basement membrane. The immunofluorescence shows granular IgG and C3. Clinically these patients present with the nephrotic syndrome.

3   Diffuse proliferative glomerulonephritis (endocapillary glomerulonephritis, post-streptococcal glomerulonephritis)

This is another example of immune complex glomerulonephritis which follows a streptococcal infection. On light-microscopy there is a general increase in the number of cells in glomerular tuft. Crescents are rare but may occasionally occur. On electron-microscopy sub-epithelial humps present in the glomerular basement membrane are diagnostic. The immunofluorescences show granular deposition of C3, IgG and properdin.

4 Diffuse extracapillary glomerulonephritis with crescents (rapidly progressive glomerulonephritis)

These changes may occur in the following conditions:
(a) Goodpasture's Syndrome;
(b) Henoch-Schönlein purpura;
(c) polyarteritis nodosa;
(d) DLE;
(e) shunt nephritis;
(f) Idiopathic crescentic nephritis.

In general these patients present with an acute fulminating form of renal failure. In Goodpasture's syndrome the renal condition may be overshadowed by the lung problems and, in Henoch–Schönlein purpura, polyarteritis nodosa, DLE and shunt nephritis, the systemic disease may predominate. The characteristic light-microscopic appearance is one of large crescents present in over 70% of glomeruli. The affected glomerular tufts are compressed to one side of Bowman's capsule by the crescents, and unlike post-streptococcal glomerulonephritis, there is little or no cellular proliferation within the tuft itself. On electron-microscopy there is disruption of the basement membrane; deposits are unusual. In Goodpasture's syndrome the immunofluorescence shows a diagnostic linear deposition of IgG, while in the others immunofluorescence with fibrin predominates in the crescent.

5 Mesangiocapillary glomerulonephritis (membrano-proliferative glomerulonephritis)

This condition manifests itself as asymptomatic proteinuria, the nephrotic syndrome or with chronic renal failure. Histologically there are two distinct types.

Type 1

This may occur idiopathically or may be associated with shunt nephritis. Light-microscopy reveals a lobular increase in mesangial matrix. Special stains show up localized thickening of the capillary walls which may become reduplicated in parts. Electron-microscopy confirms the splitting of the capillary basement membrane by the interposition of mesangial cytoplasm between the inner and outer layers giving rise to the so-called tram-tracks. On immunofluorescence there is granular deposition of IgG and C3.

Type 2

This may also be idiopathic but may occur after measles infection where it may be associated with partial lipodystrophy. (This condition is rare and is characterized by loss of subcutaneous fat over the face, upper trunk and arms). On light-microscopy there is thickening of the capillary walls due to deposits in addition to some mesangial and endothelial proliferation. Electron-microscopy confirms these dense ribbon-like deposits to be present in the centre of the glomerular basement membrane giving rise to the descriptive term 'dense deposit disease'. Immunofluorescence reveals C3 and IgM.

6   Focal proliferative glomerulonephritis

These changes occur in association with:
1   DLE;
2   polyarteritis;
3   Henoch-Schönlein purpura;
4   SBE or shunt nephritis.
   On light-microscopy there is a focal and segmental proliferation of the endothelial and epithelial cells. The electron-microscopic appearances parallel those on light-microscopy. Immunofluorescence reveals granular deposition of IgG or IgA in all cases with the exception of polyarteritis nodosa, where fibrin is usually seen. Similar light microscopic appearances are also seen in IgA nephropathy (Berger's disease), a condition characterized by recurrent episodes of haematuria. However, the diagnosis can be made on histological examination, since immunofluorescence reveals mesangial deposition of IgA spread throughout the tufts and not localized to the histologically abnormal areas.

7   Focal glomerular sclerosis or hyalinosis

This is another example of focal change of unknown aetiology. The condition presents either as asymptomatic proteinuria or as steroid-resistant nephrotic syndrome in children, and progresses inexorably to chronic renal failure. On light-microscopy there is no cellular proliferation but rather a local increase in mesangial fibrillar material starting in the tufts in the juxtamedullary region. The electron-microscopy reveals fusion of the foot processes with increase in basement membrane material. Immunofluorescence reveals granular IgM which, unlike Berger's disease, is limited to the histologically abnormal areas.

CLINICAL SYNDROMES

The glomerulonephritides can give rise to five basic clinical syndromes although, as Table 8.3 indicates, there is considerable overlap between them. This section is undoubtedly the most important of the chapter since from a practitioner's point of view this is how a patient may present. If management is to be logical, then the correct path of investigation should be undertaken and one ought to have at least some knowledge of the possible pathological process causing the syndrome.

1 Recurrent haematuria.
2 Asymptomatic proteinuria.
3 Acute nephritic syndrome.
4 Nephrotic syndrome.
5 Chronic renal failure.

Painless recurrent haematuria

Haematuria may be a symptom of disease occurring anywhere in the renal tract. Intermittent haematuria of glomerular origin, however, is usually a disease of the young, not very brisk and may not even be visible to the naked eye.

Causes

(a) Exercise haematuria.
(b) Berger's disease (mesangial IgA).
(c) Henoch Schönlein disease.
(d) Bacterial endocarditis.
(e) Connective tissue disorders—vasculitis.

Table 8.3 Basic clinical syndromes.

Clinical syndrome	Clinical feature	Possible renal histological features
Asymptomatic proteinuria	Asymptomatic, detected on urine testing only	Focal proliferative GN Focal sclerosing GN Mesangiocapillary GN
Benign recurrent haematuria	Episodes of macroscopic haematuria following intercurrent infection or exercise	Focal proliferative GN Immunofluorescence positive for IgA
Nephrotic syndrome	Proteinuria, hypoalbuminaemia and oedema	Minimal change GN Membranous GN Mesangiocapillary GN Focal sclerosis GN Focal proliferative GN
Acute renal failure	Either classical post-strep GN or acute rapidly progressive renal failure	Diffuse proliferative GN Crescentic GN (including Goodpasture's Syndrome)
Chronic renal failure	Present either de novo or as a progression from the nephrotic syndrome	Focal sclerosing GN Diffuse proliferative GN Crescentic GN Membranous GN Mesangiocapillary GN

Histologically, the glomeruli vary from normal to mild focal or diffuse proliferative changes. Perhaps the most common disorder is Berger's disease, which is associated with uniform IgA deposition in the mesangium of the glomeruli despite only focal changes on light-microscopy. This condition usually carries a good prognosis and needs to be differentiated from the more sinister vasculitic disorders, e.g. polyarteritis nodosa. Renal biopsy is the only method by which a firm diagnosis can be made.

Asymptomatic proteinuria

Asymptomatic proteinuria may be due to:
1   focal proliferative GN
   (a)   Henoch-Schönlein purpura;
   (b)   systemic lupus erythematosus (SLE);
   (c)   polyarteritis nodosa;
   (d)   bacterial endocarditis;
   (e)   Shunt nephritis.
2   focal glomerulosclerosis (focal hyalinosis).
3   mesangiocapillary glomerulonephritis.

Henoch-Schönlein Purpura

This is a disease principally of childhood (peak age of presentation three years) but which may also occur in adults. It is characterized by four features.
1   Renal involvement producing asymptomatic proteinuria (and often haematuria), the nephrotic syndrome or rapidly progressive glomerulonephritis. The severity of renal disease is parallelled by the histological change so that the asymptomatic proteinuria is associated with focal proliferative change, whereas crescentic glomerulonephritis is seen in the rapidly progressive glomerulonephritis.
2   Nonthrombocytopenic purpura which occurs on the buttocks and the extensor surfaces of the limbs. The lesions, which are usually raised, need to be differentiated from those seen in idiopathic thrombocytopenic purpura, leukaemia, meningococcal septicaemia and other vasculitides.
3   Gut involvement due to a vasculitis similar to that seen in the skin. This gives rise to colicky abdominal pain which may be asso-

ciated with rectal bleeding. Intussusception and perforation may occur.

4 Arthritis affecting particularly the knees and ankles.

The aetiology of the condition is unknown, but it often follows an upper respiratory tract infection, although the association is less clear cut than in post-streptococcal glomerulonephritis. The diagnosis is usually made on the clinical picture and is supported by the renal biopsy appearances which are additionally useful for prognostication. The serum IgA is elevated in 50% of cases but there is no change in the complement components.

There is no effective treatment for the renal disease but the skin lesion responds to corticosteroids or Dapsone. Surgical intervention may be necessary for intussusception or perforation.

Focal glomerulosclerosis

Patients present with either asymptomatic proteinuria or the nephrotic syndrome without any other features. Renal deterioration gradually occurs so that dialysis becomes necessary. The condition is unresponsive to therapy and unfortunately may recur in a transplanted kidney.

Mesangiocapillary glomerulonephritis

This may also present as asymptomatic proteinuria, the nephrotic syndrome or as chronic renal failure. Although there are two histologically distinct types their clinical courses are identical.

Type 1 (characterized by splitting of the glomerular basement membrane) may occur in shunt nephritis and where this is the case, removal of the infected focus results in improvement in renal function. The condition is associated with complement activation usually by the classic pathway.

Type 2 (dense deposit disease) may occur in association with partial lipodystrophy. The alternate pathway is involved and C3 nephritic factor may be demonstrated in plasma. Treatment with prednisolone either alone or with immunosuppressants and anticoagulants may result in slowing down the rate of renal deterioration. The patients ultimately go into renal failure.

NEPHROTIC SYNDROME

Almost all histological patterns of glomerulonephritis can be associated with the nephrotic syndrome:

1 minimal change glomerulonephritis.
2 focal glomerulosclerosis.
3 membranous glomerulonephritis.
4 mesangiocapillary glomerulonephritis.
5 focal proliferative glomerulonephritis.

Minimal-change glomerulonephritis

This is the commonest cause of the nephrotic syndrome in children where it has a peak instance between two and three years of age. It is associated with selective proteinuria (see p. 26) and carries an excellent prognosis so that spontaneous remission may occur and hypertension or deterioration in renal function are unusual. The condition may also occur in adults, but here the proteinuria may be less selective, and hypertension and renal impairment may be seen. There are no characteristic features clinically and the diagnosis is made on the basis of protein selectivity and renal biopsy appearance. The condition usually responds to steroid therapy (more so in children than in adults) so that proteinuria disappears within eight weeks of treatment. Unfortunately, however, cessation of therapy may be associated with a relapse so that a further course of steroids or cyclophosphamide may be necessary (see Chapter 9).

Membranous glomerulonephritis

This condition gives rise to the nephrotic syndrome. Where the antigen is known and its removal is possible, e.g. resection of a carcinoma, discontinuation of penicillamine, then there is histological and clinical improvement. The idiopathic variety runs a variable course. Spontaneous resolution may occur after many years of proteinuria in up to 50% of patients while, in the remainder, gradual deterioration in renal function may lead ultimately to dialysis. The diagnosis is made on the biopsy appearances (particularly the spikes seen on the thin sections stained with silver). Treatment is uncertain; although it may be possible to reduce or abolish proteinuria with corticosteroids, it is doubtful that they effect the long-term prognosis.

ACUTE RENAL FAILURE (acute nephritic syndrome)

This occurs most dramatically in post-streptococcal glomerulone-phritis, but it is also seen in rapidly progressive glomerulonephritis.

Post-streptococcal glomerulonephritis

This occurs 2–3 weeks after a streptococcal infection, usually affect-ing either the throat or the skin. Clinically there is a recrudescence of fever associated with malaise, headache, loin pain and oliguria. Hypertension is common and fluid retention may lead to pulmonary oedema so that this patient suffers from dyspnoea and swelling, particularly affecting the eyes. The urine, since it contains red cells, has a smoky appearance. The clinical picture is often suspicious but investigations will support it. A throat or wound swab will often grow the organism unless antibiotics have been given. The antistreptolysin-O (ASO) titre may also be modified if antibiotics have been given. The third component of complement is depressed during the active stage and remains low for up to 6 weeks. There may be evidence of renal impairment with a raised blood urea and crea-tinine; the urine contains red cells and protein. In general the prog-nosis is excellent; the majority recover spontaneously although a few may continue to suffer from significant proteinuria or go on to a state of chronic renal failure. Occasionally oliguria may persist so that the patient requires dialysis. The patients are managed symptomatically for their acute renal failure (see Chapter 7) and no specific therapy is indicated. Renal biopsy will only be necessary in those cases where the presentation is atypical or where renal failure persists.

Rapidly progressive glomerulonephritis

The presentation here is less dramatic than in poststreptococcal glomerulonephritis; nevertheless patients present with renal impair-ment which has come on over a matter of a few weeks. The condition may be caused by:

1 Goodpasture's syndrome;
2 acute vasculitis, e.g. polyarteritis nodosa, SLE, Henoch-Schönlein purpura;
3 idiopathic rapidly progressive glomerulonephritis.

Goodpasture's Syndrome

This rare condition results from the development of an antibody against basement membrane in both the glomeruli and the lungs. As well as suffering from renal failure, lung haemorrhages may occur and overshadow the renal disease. The diagnosis is confirmed by demonstrating either the antiglomerular basement membrane antibody or the presence of IgG deposited linearly along the basement membrane. Formerly the prognosis was invariably poor but there was some evidence to suggest that the pulmonary haemorrhage could be controlled by bilateral nephrectomy. Nowadays, the specific antibody can be removed by plasmapheresis and along with immunosuppressive therapy (steroids, cyclophosphamide) and, if necessary, dialysis, patients stand a reasonable chance of survival.

Idiopathic rapidly progressive glomerulonephritis

Histologically this is identical to Goodpasture's Syndrome except that there is no linear deposition of immunoglobulin on the basement membrane. Unfortunately recovery in renal function is rare, and therapy with corticosteroids, cyclophosphamide, Persantin and anticoagulants has been tried more in desperation than hope, usually with disappointing results.

CHRONIC RENAL FAILURE

In this syndrome gradual nephron loss has occurred, allowing adaptation to take place in the remaining nephrons. The patients may either present *de novo* or may have been followed up as their proteinuria or nephrotic syndrome has given way to renal failure. The condition may be due to:

1 focal glomerulosclerosis;
2 diffuse proliferative glomerulonephritis with or without crescent formation;
3 membranous glomerulonephritis;
4 mesangiocapillary glomerulonephritis.

In some instances the disease process responsible for the syndrome cannot be ascertained, since renal histology merely shows massive destruction of glomeruli with tubular atrophy. In general, by the time a patient has reached this stage, conservative therapy is ineffectual.

Chapter 9
Nephrotic Syndrome

This is a clinical syndrome which includes as its features heavy proteinuria ($>3.5\,\mathrm{gm}^{-2}$) with a low plasma albumin and severe dependent oedema. Hypercholesterolaemia is often present as well.

Incidence

It is 2–3 times more common in children than in adults; the peak incidence is between two and three years of age. It occurs in male children 2.5 times more than in females—in adults, there is equal incidence in both sexes. Neonatal nephrotic syndrome occurs but is very rare.

Causes

1 Primary glomerulonephritis
   minimal-change GN
   membranous GN
   membrano-proliferative GN or mesangiocapillary glomerulo-nephritis (MCGN)
   focal glomerulosclerosis
   focal proliferative GN
2 Secondary glomerulonephritis
   SLE
   Henoch-Schönlein purpura
   carcinoma of bronchus
   Hodgkins lymphoma, etc.
3 Metabolic diseases
   diabetes mellitus
   amyloid disease (myelomatosis)
4 Infection
   malaria, syphilis, leprosy,
   Staph. albus. Hepatitis B.

5 Drug-induced GN
    penicillamine, gold, Tridione,
    phenytoin, captopril, etc.
6 Cardiovascular
    constrictive pericarditis
    renal vein thrombosis
7 Bee and insect stings

Clinical picture

In children the onset may be abrupt and sometimes follows upper respiratory infection. Peri-orbital oedema may be the presenting feature but ascites and leg oedema may also be present.

The onset in adults is often insidious, with gradual development of pitting oedema. The lower half of the body becomes grossly swollen with genital involvement, ascites and later pleural effusions may develop. The patient may notice that his urine is frothy.

Renal function

This is usually normal, although (rarely) oliguric renal failure may rapidly develop.

Creatinine clearances may be inappropriately high.

Plasma proteins

Plasma albumin is low but α_2 globulins and fibrinogen levels are elevated. γ globulins tend to be low and might account for the tendency to infection.

Urinary proteins

Heavy proteinuria (greater than 5 g day^{-1} in adults) will be present. Hyaline casts and fat bodies may be seen in the urine on microscopy. The presence of red blood corpuscles might indicate MCGN or proliferative GN.

Blood coagulation

Platelet count, plasma fibrinogen and factor VIII may be raised and these can lead to a state of potential hypercoagulability. This may be aggravated by haemoconcentration.

Blood volume

This is low when plasma albumin levels fall, due to reduction in plasma oncotic pressure.

Blood pressure is usually normal.

Plasma lipids

Hypercholesterolaemia is common in the nephrotic syndrome and the plasma levels are inversely proportional to the plasma albumin levels. Plasma triglycerides may also be raised.

The cause of hypercholesterolaemia is not known but may be related to mobilization of fat in order to synthesize protein.

Plasma calcium

Levels of plasma calcium tend to be low in the nephrotic syndrome, possibly because of the associated hypoalbuminaemia and diminished absorption by the intestine. Urinary calcium losses are extremely low.

Urinary electrolytes

Because of marked secondary hyperaldosteronism, intense sodium retention occurs, and this is evidenced by a very low urinary sodium concentration. On the other hand, urinary potassium losses are high.

Differential protein clearance

The ratio of the clearance of albumin (or transferrin) to that of IgG gives a useful selectivity index in childhood nephrotic syndrome. A highly selective index (<0.2) would be in favour of minimal-change glomerulonephritis which should be steroid responsive. This is useful in paediatrics, for renal biopsy might be avoided.

Pathophysiology

The underlying glomerular abnormality in the majority of children suffering from the nephrotic syndrome is very slight. Light-microscopically, no abnormality can be seen and no abnormal deposits of immunoglobulins or complement can be seen on immunofluorescence. By electron-microscopy, however, fusion of epithelial foot processes will be observed.

Nearly all other forms of nephrotic syndrome are associated with morphological changes characteristic of one type of glomerulonephritis or another, e.g. membranous deposits, proliferations of cells, crescents, eosinophilic or amyloid deposits.

Where the nephrotic syndrome is considered to be due to constrictive pericarditis or to renal vein thrombosis, the glomerular appearances are non-specific and may include basement membrane thickening and interstitial oedema.

Nevertheless, in the majority of cases, some form of damage to the glomerular basement membrane is the primary factor in the development of the syndrome. The consequent loss of protein from the body in addition to the amount that can be replaced by hepatic synthesis leads inevitably to a lowering of the plasma protein concentration, with the result that salt and water are retained and redistributed in the extravascular compartment (see Fig. 9.1).

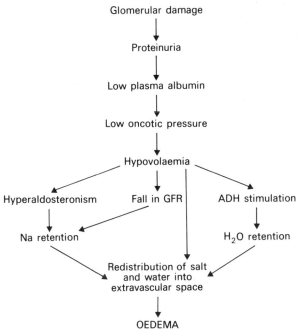

Fig. 9.1 Mechanisms for development of oedema.

Investigations

The intensity of investigations will depend largely upon the patient's age.

Under the age of five years, 85% of nephrotics have minimal-change lesions. Over the age of 11 years only 20–30% will be due to this condition. It is, therefore, accepted that renal biopsy is not a necessary first-line investigation in those under ten years.

Full clinical history and examination are necessary in all patients. Urine microscopy and 24-hour urinary protein measurement are essential.

An assessment of glomerular filtration rate (by creatinine clearance or Cr_{51} EDTA clearance) should be performed and plasma proteins should be measured. Differential protein index may help in the case of children (this gives an indication of the size of protein molecules being excreted). Serum complement activity and immune complex concentration should be measured.

In children with haematuria, hypertension, reduced renal function, low complement levels and where the proteinuria is non-selective, a renal biopsy is clearly indicated. *All* adult nephrotics should be biopsied.

Complications of nephrotic syndrome

(a) *Protein malnutrition* leading to muscle wasting, striae, osteoporosis and loss of hair.

(b) *Infections*—cutaneous
            —primary pneumococcal peritonitis
            —urinary tract infections
            —septicaemias
due to low gammaglobulins and loss of cell-mediated responses.

(c) *Tendency to thrombosis*
  (i) due to increased factor VIII, fibrinogen and platelets;
  (ii) hypovolaemia.

(d) Ischaemic heart disease? due to hyperlipidaemia.

(e) Acute hypovolaemia—may precipitate acute renal failure.

General management

Control of oedema
  Diuretics and potassium conservation
  Restore plasma protein by i.v. infusion

Diet
  Normal diet containing at least 70 g protein
  Low sodium (approx 50 mmol day^{-1})

Infections
  Antibiotics

Coagulation
  Treat venous thrombosis with anticoagulants
  The role of prophylactic anticoagulants is uncertain

Specific treatment

Minimal-Change GN

Condition may be self limiting and no treatment is necessary unless oedema is present.

Corticosteroids

Prednisone or prednisolone up to 60 mg per m^2 per day for one month. Gradually reduce during second month.

Rapid remission will occur in most children in under one month. Should continue for two months before labelling anyone as steroid resistant.

50% remain in long remission (> 1 year). The rest may relapse after viral infections. Further courses of steroids can be given though not without risk of complications. Minimum effective dose should be found for each patient and alternate-day therapy tried.

Cyclophosphamide

Can induce long and stable remissions in steroid-dependent nephrotics: dose 3 mg per kg bodyweight per day for eight weeks.

Leucopaenia unusual at this dose but weekly leucocyte counts should be done. Alopecia is unusual at this dose, but amenorrhoea and oligospermia may be long-term hazards from prolonged courses of therapy.

Azathioprine

This has not been found to be of value except in those cases associated with SLE.

Chlorambucil

This may well be as effective as cyclosphosphamide in the long-term.

Disadvantages of long-term steroid therapy

1 Cushingoid habitus.
2 Hirsutism.
3 Osteoporosis and avascular necrosis.
4 Susceptibility to infections.
5 Hypercoagulability of blood leads to venous thrombosis.
6 Growth retardation in children.
7 Cataracts.
8 Peptic ulceration.
9 Diabetes mellitus.
10 Steroid psychosis.

Prognosis in nephrotic syndrome

In children with minimal-change glomerulonephritis, long-term re-missions carry a favourable long-term prognosis and, even in those resistant to steroids, after cyclophosphamide treatment, approximately 40% will have a relapse-free course over ten years. Children who are resistant both to steroids and cyclophosphamide carry a prognosis which is dependent upon the degree of renal damage plus the inherent dangers of the syndrome itself.

A similar situation pertains to adults. The underlying disease process is the major deciding factor. In the case of infection-induced or drug-induced nephrotic syndrome there is always the theoretical possibility of remission following the removal of the original insulting agent. In certain malignant syndromes, e.g. bronchial carcinoma or Hodgkin's disease, treatment of the malignancy may lead to remission of the nephrotic syndrome. Hypersensitivity reactions such as bee stings carry a good prognosis.

In SLE the outcome depends upon the degree of glomerular and systemic involvement but, as a rule with steroids and azathioprine, long remissions are certainly possible.

Where secondary amyloid is responsible, improvement would be expected if the initial stimulating factor was removed, e.g. bronchiectatic lung, empyema or osteomyelitis, but unfortunately many patients with amyloid have a primary cause that is difficult to eradicate, e.g. rheumatoid arthritis, ankylosing spondylitis and myeloma.

As the glomerular lesions causing the nephrotic syndrome progress, the degree of proteinuria may diminish with the falling GFR — thus making it easier to control oedema and hypovolaemia.

Undoubtedly, many nephrotics who eventually reach a stage of chronic renal failure will be taken on to dialysis and transplant programmes.

Chapter 10
Urinary Tract Infections

Whereas urinary tract symptoms are very common in adult females, it is now appreciated that the major damage to kidneys occurs in infancy and childhood.

The prevention of damage by infection to growing kidneys is therefore of great importance if subsequent renal failure in early adulthood is to be avoided.

PROBLEMS IN CHILDHOOD

Presentation

The younger the child, the less specific will be the presenting symptoms. Below the age of two years, failure to thrive, jaundice, feeding problems, screaming attacks, diarrhoea, vomiting and fever are the most common symptoms.

Urinary frequency, dysuria, abdominal and loin pains become more common as the child grows and is better able to express himself.

In the newborn baby, urinary infection can easily be missed. Check for weight loss, the presence of jaundice, character of urinary stream (in males) and bowel habit. Examination should include neurological examination to exclude spinal cord lesions which can lead to a neurogenic bladder. Always feel for an enlarged bladder. A family history of urinary tract problems may be relevant.

Infecting organisms

Usually gut flora invade the perineum and ascend into and colonize the bladder. In neonatal children, blood-borne organisms may be important (possibly also important *in utero*). 75% of children who have urinary tract infections will have a recurrence within 2 years.

Factors which predispose to recurrent urinary infections

1 Mechanical obstruction, e.g. urethral valves.
2 Vesicoureteric reflux.
3 Neurological abnormalities leading to bladder dysfunction, e.g. spina bifida.
4 Bladder diverticula.
5 Calculi.
6 Incomplete bladder emptying, constipation.
7 Impaired immune responses.

Diagnosis

It is always important to establish that organisms are present and multiplying in the urinary tract before treatment is started. Quantitative estimation of colony counts in a freshly voided sample of urine must, therefore, be performed. Collection of urine in children can be very difficult and great skill on the part of nursing staff and parents is called for.

(a) Clean catch or midstream samples may be obtained after first cleansing the vulva or penis with soap and water.
(b) In small infants sterile plastic bags can be applied to the clean perineum. As soon as urine is passed, the bag should be removed and the urine cultured.
(c) Suprapubic aspiration of the full bladder is a useful technique.
(d) Dip slide held in urinary stream.
(e) Catheter specimens may be obtained only if all other methods have failed.

Cultures

The freshly voided urine should be taken to the laboratory and processed without delay. If delays are inevitable, the urine can be kept in a refrigerator for up to 48 hours: if left at room temperature for more than two hours, erroneous bacterial counts will be obtained. Dip slide cultures will avoid this problem and can be posted to a laboratory from a domiciliary practice. *Escherichia coli* is the usual offending organism in girls and is present in 80-90% of all urinary infections. In boys it is present in only about 50%, followed closely by proteus species.

Bacterial counts

Quantitative bacterial counts of over 10^5 ml^{-1} is considered to represent significant infection in urethral and catheter specimens of urine. In suprapubic samples, any growth at all is considered significant. The presence of more than one organism suggests contamination from urethral and perineal organisms. The test should be repeated.

Pus cells

The presence of pus cells in concentrations of greater than 10 mm^{-3} of uncentrifuged fresh urine indicates inflammation of the urinary tract. It should be remembered that their presence may not always indicate significant urinary infection, whereas their absence does not always exclude significant infection.

Further investigations

The presence of urinary infection in an infant should always be taken seriously. The likelihood is that scarring of the kidney occurs only in children under the age of four years. The damage might even have been done before the diagnosis of the first infection is made. The patterns of investigations therefore will be determined according to the value that each is expected to provide.

The use of the plain abdominal X-ray and ultrasound will provide fairly accurate information regarding stones, bladder emptying and reflux but may be unreliable in demonstrating renal scars. DMSA scans will identify scars very accurately and DTPA scans provide information regarding obstruction and reflux. In the very young (under 6 months) the micturating cysto-urethrogram should always be performed first but in older children this unpleasant investigation can often be avoided. The intravenous urogram can thus be used as a confirmatory test rather than a primary investigation.

Approximately half the children investigated along these lines will show anatomical abnormalities of the urinary tract. The majority will have vesicoureteric reflux with or without scarring of the renal cortex. Others will have duplex or horseshoe kidneys, stones or ureterocoeles.

Acute infections

(a) General measures:
high fluid intake;
frequent voiding.
(b) Specific measures:
culture urine and examine microscopically;
start 'best bet' antimicrobial drug;
reassess antibiotic when sensitivity of the organisms is known;
if no improvement is obvious after 48 hours change antibiotic;
continue antibiotic for 7–10 days;
culture urine 48 hours after completing antibiotic course.

Best-bet antimicrobial drugs

1 Cotrimoxazole (Septrin) or Trimethoprim
2 Ampicillin or amoxycillin
3 Augmentin

If the child is very ill, it probably has an accompanying septicaemia and will require parenteral therapy with Gentamicin, amoxycillin or cephoxatime. Care should be taken in treating the newborn with sulphonamide-containing drugs, they may interfere with the bilirubin binding to protein.

Vesico ureteric reflux

This is the commonest cause of recurrent urinary tract infection in childhood.

Causes

(a) Developmental abnormality of ureterovesical junction resulting in a short intramural course through the bladder wall (Fig. 10.1).
(b) Association with ureterocoeles or renal ectopia.
(c) Bladder neck obstruction or neuropathic bladder.
(d) Trauma due to stones, infections, etc.
During bladder filling or during voiding, when intravesical pressure rises, retrograde flow of urine up the ureter will occur. This may be classified according to its severity (Fig. 10.2).

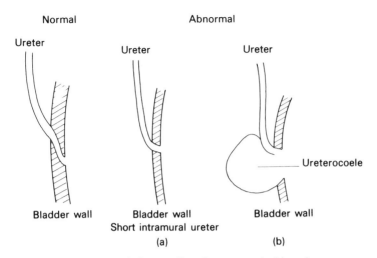

Fig. 10.1 Developmental abnormality of ureterovesical junction.

Reflux predisposes to recurrent infection because it leads to urinary retention, allows reflux of infected urine into the upper renal tract and it may have a direct mechanical effect on the renal medulla, particularly when intrarenal reflux occurs.

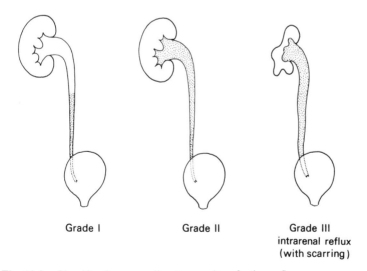

Fig. 10.2 Classification according to severity of urine reflux.

Renal scarring

It is thought that scarring of the kidneys only occurs in children and it is almost always associated with vesicoureteric reflux. Up to 20% of all children who have had symptomatic urinary infection have been found to have scarred kidneys. On intravenous urography, scars occur opposite deformed calyces and are recognized by a reduction in cortical width. The adjacent renal tissue grows normally thus accentuating the appearance of the scar. Polar calyces seem to be more susceptible to the effects of severe reflux than the more centrally placed ones.

Vesicoureteric reflux in children can lead to reflux nephropathy with hypertension and renal failure. Early detection and treatment are, therefore, important.

Management

1 Exclude obstruction to lower urinary tract. If present, this should be treated urgently by surgery.
2 Control of infection. Acute infections should be treated with 3- to 5-day courses of appropriate antibiotics. Long-term treatment can best be achieved by antibiotics in low dosage, e.g. Co-trimoxazole 1 tablet nightly or nitrofurantoin 50 mg nightly after a full eradicating course.

This prophylaxis should probably be continued for as long as reflux persists and until the kidneys are fully grown. In addition, the child should be trained to drink plenty of fluid, to empty the bladder frequently, to perform double micturition at least once per day (preferably at night) and to avoid constipation. Periodic urinary cultures and assessment of renal function should be performed. Many refluxing ureters will stop spontaneously only to start again if further infection occurs. The careful control of infection is therefore important so that ureteric re-implantation rarely is necessary.

URINARY TRACT INFECTIONS IN ADULTS

Dysuria is a common symptom in adult females and accounts for about 1 in every 100 general practice consultations. Symptoms are most common during the sexually active years; though they may be severe and recurrent, they rarely lead to renal failure.

Once the kidneys have grown normally to adult size, recurrent infections rarely threaten life unless obstruction, stones or neurological complications occur. Nevertheless, recurrent urinary infections in the adult call for thorough investigation in order to establish the size and configuration of the kidneys and urogenital tract and to exclude surgically correctable conditions. Young males are rarely affected by urinary infections. If they are, a search should be made for stones, a history of gout, prostatitis or neurological disorders.

Clinical syndromes

1   Frequency and dysuria

This is a syndrome that occurs almost exclusively in women and is characterized by painful burning micturition, suprapubic pain and strangury. In approximately half the patients, pyuria and bacteriuria will be found and these would be expected to respond to a short course of antibiotics, e.g. Trimethoprim 200 mg b.d. or Ampicillin 250 mg q.d.s. Failure to respond to treatment would indicate:

(a)   the wrong choice of drug;
(b)   inadequate dosage or duration of treatment;
(c)   the development of bacterial resistance; or
(d)   anatomical abnormalities and stones.

In the non-bacterial cases (this is sometimes called the 'urethral syndrome') the cause of symptoms is often difficult to assess. In some patients symptoms may be precipitated by sexual intercourse, in others wearing tight undergarments, the use of deodorants, bathing detergents and voluntary withholding of micturition may have aetiological significance. A high fluid intake, frequent voiding, particularly after intercourse, avoiding detergents, etc., may prevent further symptoms, but in some cases post-intercourse antibiotics such as trimethoprim or nitrofurantoin may be helpful.

Fastidious organisms such as clamydia may be present in the lower urinary tract but will be missed unless special culture techniques are used. These organisms usually require prolonged courses of antibiotics such as Erythromycin for their eradication. Sterile pyuria should always alert one to the possibility of tuberculous infection of the renal tract. Three early morning urine specimens should be sent for special culture.

2 Acute pyelonephritis

Loin pain and fever often associated with rigors are the commonest presenting symptoms. Lower urinary tract symptoms (frequency and dysuria) are not necessarily present though patients may complain that their urine appears cloudy and smells strongly. Examination reveals tenderness over the renal angles, sometimes with spasm of the spinalis muscles. The urine may contain numerous pus cells and bacteria and blood cultures may be positive.

3 Asymptomatic bacteriuria

This can only be discovered by routine testing or during epidemiological screening.

The most important adult worth screening is the pregnant patient. It has been shown that 3-7% of all pregnant patients at booking clinics have asymptomatic bacteriuria and if these infections are not treated, 20% will develop acute pyelonephritis during pregnancy. If followed up six months after pregnancy, approximately one-third will have radiological abnormalities, and one-quarter may get recurrent or persistent bacteriuria.

4 Interstitial nephritis

This is the term used to describe a pathological process in which infection plays a relatively minor role.

Causes of interstitial nephritis:
(a)   analgesic abuse;
(b)   ischaemia due to hypertension, sickle-cell disease;
(c)   heavy metal poisoning, e.g. lead, cadmium;
(d)   metabolic causes, e.g. hypercalcaemia, hyperuricaemia and oxalosis;
(e)   drug reactions, e.g. methicillin, sulphonamides, phenindione, rifampicin;
(f)   vesicoureteric reflux with infection;
(g)   congenital dysplasia;
(h)   radiation damage;
(i)   endemic (Balkan) nephropathy.

The gross appearance of these kidneys is very similar, though papillary necrosis is likely to be attributed to analgesic abuse, sickle-cell disease or diabetes mellitus. The histological appearances of interstitial oedema, cellular infiltration, fibrosis, tubular atrophy and ischaemia are common to them all. It should be remembered that urinary tract infection often occurs secondarily.

5 Chronic pyelonephritis

The appearance of shrinkage and scarring of the kidney cortex as seen radiologically in patients who have had recurrent urinary infections since childhood is known as chronic pyelonephritis. These patients usually are hypertensive and have impaired renal function. It is a progressive condition which can end in renal failure.

Important factors contributing to urinary tract infection

Normally the lower urinary tract is protected against local invasion of bacteria from the perineum by:
(a) the hydrokinetic effect of repeated bladder emptying; and
(b) the antibacterial effect of the secretory IgA produced by the bladder mucosal cells. Furthermore a competent ureterovesical valve mechanism will protect against bacterial invasion up the ureters.

Failure of any of these mechanisms will render the individual susceptible to urinary tract infections, which in the female is facilitated by the short urethra, urethral trauma during intercourse and retrograde flow up the urethra both during micturition and bathing.

If as a result of reflux, bacteria reach the medullary tissue, they will proliferate in an area where there is high osmolality, a high ammonia concentration and consequently poor phagocyte function. Furthermore the persistence of L forms is encouraged. Reflux has been shown to occur only into compound papillae; normal-shaped papillae are protected by virtue of the angle at which the ducts open on to its surface.

BACTERIOLOGICAL DIAGNOSIS

Culture of freshly voided midstream urine (MSU) is essential.
(a) Cleaning of vulva or glans with soap and water.
(b) Part the labia in the female.

(c)   Collect MSU in wide-necked jar (female); collect MSU in universal container (male).

(d)   Send sample to laboratory immediately (if delayed, keep in 4°C fridge).

(e)   Inoculate dip slide or culture plate.

The dip slide can be held in the urinary stream and sent to the laboratory for incubation, or can be incubated in the GP's surgery.

A significant infection is assumed if a pure growth of more than $100\,000$ colonies ml^{-1} is found. Organism counts of $10\,000\,ml^{-1}$ or less represent urethral contamination particularly if the growth is mixed. Counts between $10\,000$ and $100\,000\,ml^{-1}$ probably warrant re-examination.

False positive cultures may well result from delay in transmitting the urine to the laboratory or delay in plating out. The processing should be completed in under two hours otherwise the specimen should be refrigerated.

Ideally, early-morning urine specimens should be cultured, for then the urine is at its most concentrated. A falsely low bacterial count may be obtained if urine is collected during a period of diuresis.

By far the most common organism seen in general practice is *Escherichia coli*, the serotypes correspond to those found in the individual's own gut. *Staphylococcus albus*, *Proteus* species and *Streptococcus faecalis* account for most of the remaining organisms. In hospital practice *Proteus*, *Strep. faecalis* and *Klebsiella* account for a significant proportion of urinary infections. *Pseudomonas pyocyanea* is mainly found in catheterized patients and in those who have been given broad-spectrum antibiotics.

Management

General measures

Many patients with symptoms suggestive of urinary tract infection will benefit from basic advice regarding proper emptying of the bladder, drinking plenty of fluid and perineal hygiene including post coital micturition. They, should also probably avoid detergents whilst bathing.

Treatment of symptomatic infections
First, urine should be taken for culture.

These patients may be very toxic, with considerable pain, fever, often vomiting and dehydrated. A high fluid intake is important and antibiotics should be started before the results of culture are known. 'Best Bet' antibiotics under these circumstances would be Amoxycillin or Ampicillin 500 mg 6-hourly or Trimethoprim 200 mg b.d. These drugs may be given intravenously if necessary. The duration of treatment is controversial but it probably need not be extended beyond 5 days.

If the choice of antibiotic has been incorrect as judged by the culture and sensitivity result (and by the patient's lack of response to treatment), the correct antibiotic should be substituted.

Careful follow-up of these patients is important for infections tend to recur fairly frequently. Relapsing infections occur in approximately one-quarter of cases and are due to inadequate treatment. Re-infections, which usually occur after an interval of 6 weeks or so are much commoner and usually denote a defect in the patient's defence mechanisms against infection. These people will often require long-term low dose prophylactic antibiotics, e.g. Trimethoprim or Cotrimoxazole 1 tablet nightly for 6-12 months.

All patients with re-infections should be fully investigated. This will include:
(a) straight abdominal X-ray for stones;
(b) ultrasound examination of kidneys and bladder;
(c) DMSA scan for renal scars;
(d) DTPA scan for evidence of obstruction or reflux;
(e) creatinine clearance and estimation of electrolytes and serum calcium.

If a surgically correctible condition is found, e.g. stones, bladder diverticulum, obstruction, etc., the appropriate measures should be undertaken under antibiotic cover. It is debatable whether vesicoureteric reflux should be corrected in the adult, but where infections are impossible to control, there may be an argument for doing so.

In the presence of a normal urinary tract, renal function and blood pressure, the patient should be heavily reassured for the dangers of progressing to chronic renal failure are extremely rare. Basic principles such as adequate fluid intake and complete voiding should be re-emphasized and prophylactic antibiotics used when indicated.

Chapter 11
Connective Tissue Disorders and the Kidney

SYSTEMIC LUPUS ERYTHEMATOSUS

Systemic lupus erythematosis (SLE) is a multisystem disease of unknown aetiology which is nine times more common in women than in men and affects them during child-bearing years. It is characterized by circulating humoral antibodies, particularly against nuclear components, and it seems likely that antibody-antigen complexes are the initiating factor in causing tissue damage.

Pathological features

SLE produces a range of glomerulonephritic changes which fall into one of three broad groups.

1 Focal proliferative glomerulonephritis indistinguishable from other forms of focal proliferation such as Henoch-Schönlein purpura or sub-acute bacterial endocarditis. Occurs in 30%. Occasionally only mild, minimal or mesangial change is apparent.

2 Membranous glomerulonephritis indistinguishable from other forms may be seen in 15%.

3 Diffuse proliferative changes occasionally severe enough to cause crescent formation are seen in 55%.

Haematoxyphil bodies, which are fragments of degenerating nuclear material, and *wire loop lesions*, which are areas of localized thickening of the capillary loops, are diagnostic of lupus nephropathy but unfortunately are found only in a minority of patients.

Clinical features

SLE affects virtually every system as follows.

Joints: arthritis and arthralgia.

Skin: butterfly rash and discoid lupus.

95

Cardiovascular system: pericarditis, myocarditis and non-bacterial endocarditis (Libman–Sacks).

Respiratory system: pleural effusion and pulmonary infiltrates.

Nervous system: cerebral lupus, transverse myelitis, lesions of the cranial nerves and retinal changes.

Haemopoietic system: anaemia, leucopenia, thrombotycopenia and circulating anticoagulants.

Renal involvement occurs in over 50% of patients although it may be a presenting feature in only 25%.

The renal disease may be manifest by:
(a)   asymptomatic proteinuria;
(b)   the nephrotic syndrome;
(c)   renal failure.

In general, those with the most marked histological abnormality, i.e. generalized proliferative glomerulonephritis, are more likely to have haematuria, to be hypertensive and to progress to renal failure. Those with membranous change are likely to have a high urinary protein loss and to have the features of the nephrotic syndrome.

Results of investigations

(a)   Anaemia.
(b)   Coombs' test often positive.
(c)   Erythrocyte sedimentation rate (ESR) raised.
(d)   Leucopenia.
(e)   ANF strongly positive (with the possible exception of patients who are uraemic).
(f)   Antibody against double-stranded DNA, i.e. DNA binding assay positive (the level of DNA binding is a poor indicator of disease activity but a sudden rise may herald an exacerbation in a patient whose disease process is quiescent).
(g)   Evidence of a complement activation with a low plasma C3 especially in patients with membranous or diffuse proliferative changes.

Management

The prognosis in lupus nephritis is probably much better than was previously feared. Although death from renal failure may occur, cerebral lupus and sepsis occurring as a complication of treatment seems to be more important. Generally, the younger the patient the better the prognosis. Prednisolone together with an immunosuppressant (usually azathioprine) remain the mainstay of treatment. It seems likely that this therapy is capable of modifying the histological appearance so that those with diffuse proliferative changes may, after a period of treatment, develop changes of membranous nephritis. High-dose parenteral methylprednisolone, plasmapheresis or the addition of anticoagulants and Persantin to steroids and Imuran have all been advocated, but their place in the management remains to be fully elucidated. The management of nephrotic syndrome or renal failure in patients with lupus nephritis is otherwise the same as previously outlined.

POLYARTERITIS NODOSA (PAN)

PAN is a condition of unknown aetiology which is slightly more common in men and occurs in patients between the ages of 20 and 40. It is characterized by focal inflammation and necrosis of the walls of medium and small arteries. There is resultant ischaemic damage to viscera of thorax and abdomen, the brain, spinal cord, peripheral nerves and muscles. The affected vessels become weakened leading to multiple aneurysms 5-10 mm in diameter. Hepatitis B antigen may be present in the blood and it is possible that the condition results from deposition of antigen–antibody complexes in the vessels, the antigen being viral in origin.

Pathological lesions

Two different lesions are seen in the kidney either alone or in combination:
1 renal polyarteritis;
2 glomerulitis.

Renal polyarteritis is the more common and affects the arcuate and interlobular arteries. There is fibrinoid necrosis and inflammation of all layers of the arterial wall and the resultant weakening may lead to multiple small aneurysms. The glomerulitis occurs in 30% of cases. The affected glomeruli show microthrombi, hypercellularity, fibrinoid necrosis and crescent formation. As the lesions heal there is fibrosis and hyalinization of the glomerular tuft.

Clinical features

Patients usually have non-specific symptoms and signs of tachycardia, anorexia, fever, weight loss, myalgia and arthralgia. In addition the following systems may be involved.

Cardiovascular system: pericarditis, myocardial ischaemia or infarction.

Respiratory system: pleurisy, bronchospasm, pulmonary infiltrates which may cavitate.

Gastrointestinal symptoms: abdominal pain, nausea, vomiting, diarrhoea with blood.

Nervous system: mononeuritis multiplex.

The clinical features of renal disease in PAN are non-specific. Inevitable renal impairment leading to renal failure occurs but the length of time taken for this to happen may vary enormously. Hypertension occurs, usually late, probably as the result of damage occurring to the glomeruli as part of the healing process. Urine contains red cells, casts and protein; the proteinuria is not usually enough to lead to the nephrotic syndrome.

Investigations

There are no diagnostic blood tests for this condition. There is often an anaemia with a raised ESR and in 80% of cases there is a leucocytosis. In those with lung involvement there is often eosinophilia. Arteriography of the renal arteries or of coeliac axis may reveal multiple aneurysms which are diagnostic of the condition. The histological picture of the kidneys in patients where there is only a glomerulonephritis is non-specific and is the same as that seen in other forms of rapidly progressive GN (see p. 66). An appearance of polyarteritis, however, is diagnostic.

Management

If left untreated, the arterial lesions lead to progressive destruction of vital organs with death from renal failure, myocardial infarction, etc. Corticosteroids in the form of prednisolone 40-60 mg a day produce rapid symptomatic relief and, if given early enough, may lead to improvement in histological changes and renal function. It is difficult to be certain, however, whether corticosteroids materially alter the long-term prognosis.

WEGENER'S GRANULOMATOSUS

This is a condition related to PAN where there is a vasculitis especially affecting the smaller vessels, but also extending to include the veins associated with a destructive sinusitis with granulomatous lesions of the nasal mucosa and pulmonary tissue. Its aetiology remains unknown.

Pathological lesion

Wegener's gramulomatosus is characterized by a focal necrotizing glomerulonephritis with haemorrhage and fibrin deposition. The histological picture is not diagnostic.

Clinical features

Wegener's granulomatatosus is characterized by similar non-specific features to those that occur in polyarteritis nodosa, namely fever, malaise, tachycardia, etc. In addition, the upper airway disease gives rise to pain, nasal discharge and even destruction of the nasal septum resulting in collapse of the bridge of the nose. A lower airway involvement gives rise to cough, haemoptysis, dyspnoea and chest pain. Radiographs may show pulmonary infiltrates which cavitate. Clinically the renal disease results in rapidly progressive renal failure. The urine contains microscopic blood, casts and protein.

Investigations

There are no diagnostic blood tests for this condition. There is an anaemia with a raised ESR and leucocytosis but, despite the lung lesions, there is no eosinophilia. The diagnosis is made by the renal histological appearances in the presence of upper and lower airways disease.

Management

Wegener's granulomatosus seems to be more amenable to treatment than polyarteritis nodosa. Prednisolone and an immunosuppressant such as Cyclophosphamide are capable of totally suppressing the disease process which is often self limiting. Once the disease has been brought into remission, therapy should be continued for a couple of years but at the end of this time it may be possible to discontinue it.

SYSTEMIC SCLEROSIS

Systemic sclerosis is a condition of unknown aetiology which is three times more common in females, affecting those between the ages of 35 and 55. The condition affects blood vessels and connective tissue leading to vascular insufficiency.

Pathological lesion

There is altered vascular reactivity of the renal blood vessels so that intense vasospasm occurs in response to cold. Histologically there is proliferation of the intimal cells with mucoid deposition. The inter-lobular arteries become severely narrowed leading to fibrinoid necrosis. In general, these changes occur predominantly in the renal cortex.

Clinical features

There are non-specific features of systemic sclerosis in the form of weakness, weight loss and diffuse muscle and skeletal stiffness. Virtually every system of the body is affected as follows.

Skin: telangiectasis, thickening and tightness of the skin particularly affecting the fingers and around the mouth. Raynaud's phenomenon.

Musculoskeletal system: pain affecting particularly the small joints. This progresses to erosive change leading to deformity. Muscle wasting also occurs.

Gastrointestinal symptoms: Systemic sclerosis in the gut leads to dysphagia, heartburn, vomiting, abdominal pain, malabsorption and bowel change. The condition may be associated with primary biliary sclerosis.

Heart and lungs: fibrosis of the lungs leads to shortness of breath. Scleroderma of the heart may occur but it is ususual.

Renal involvement manifests itself by proteinuria, hypertension and uraemia. Proteinuria is often mild and may be present for years without progressing. The urine may contain a few red cells but does not contain casts. Hypertension may be paroxysmal or continuous and is probably related to vasospasm initially, but later to permanent renal artery change leading to increased renin production. In a minority hypertension and oliguric renal failure may develop suddenly.

Investigations

There are no diagnostic blood tests for this condition. The ESR is usually raised and the antinuclear factor (ANF) and rheumatoid factor may be positive. The diagnosis is made on the clinical picture.

Management

Systemic sclerosis is a progressive condition which does not respond to any form of treatment; corticosteroids are totally ineffective. Renal involvement should be managed by aggressive treatment of hypertension with haemodialysis if anuria occurs. In the past bilateral nephrectomy has been advocated as the only way of controlling this condition but more recent evidence suggests that this may not be necessary. The prognosis remains poor but patients have been treated with long-term haemodialysis and even transplantation with some degree of success.

Chapter 12
Metabolic Conditions and the Kidney

DIABETES MELLITUS

Most renal problems in patients with diabetes mellitus are the result of glomerulosclerosis. The histological appearances of this are, for convenience, divided into descriptive groups although they probably represent differing degrees of renal involvement.

1 Nodular

This form, which was described by Kimmelstiee and Wilson, is pathognomonic of diabetes. It consists of homogeneous eosinophilic spherical masses arising from the intercapillary tissue (or 'mesangium' *q.v.*) in the centres of one or more of the peripheral glomerular lobules.

2 Diffuse glomerular lesions

These changes are twice as common as the nodular form which is only seen where diffuse changes are present. It is arguable whether the two are the result of different pathogenetic processes, or the nodular form represents a worsening of the diffuse process. The diffuse lesions start as an increase in the mesangial matrix and a diffuse thickening of the capillary walls on the glomerular tufts. As it worsens all capillaries are affected so that their lumina are reduced and ultimately obliterated leading to hyalinization of glomerular tissue. These changes are relatively non-specific and it may be impossible to distinguish them from changes seen in membranous glomerulonephritis or amyloid. Their importance is that they occur early in the disease and their severity correlates with the severity of clinical disease.

3 Exudative lesion (acellular hyaline, fibrin cap, capsular drop, hyaline-fibrinoid)

This is the least specific of the changes. Microscopically it consists of eosinophilic spherical deposits found either moulded over a capillary loop or attached to the inside of Bowman's capsule. These deposits probably occur as a late result of fibrosis and hyalinization.

4 Vascular lesions

Arteries in the kidney show atherosclerotic changes which are more advanced than would be expected for the patient's age. The arterioles also become sclerotic and involvement of the efferent arteriole is specific for diabetes.

5 Tubular lesions

These are non-specific changes resulting from ischaemia or infection and appear as tubular atrophy with surrounding areas of fibrosis and cellular infiltration.

Electron microscopy

The changes seen on electron microscopy are:
(a)   thickening of the glomerular capillary basement membrane;
(b)   deposition of basement-membrane-like material and fibrin in the mesangium.

Pathogenesis

Diabetic nephropathy and retinopathy both result from microangiopathy and their development is related, certainly, to the duration of diabetes mellitus and also, probably, to the degree of diabetic control. In general, it is those who develop diabetes mellitus before the age of 20 who progress to renal problems, since patients who are older at the time of diagnosis are more likely to die from cerebrovascular and cardiovascular disease.

The pathogenesis of these diabetic glomerular changes remains uncertain but it seems likely that the carbohydrate content and the glucopeptides to which it is bound are changed.

Clinical features

Although histological changes are common even at an early stage in diabetes, clinical disease is relatively less so. Proteinuria is the first sign of diabetic renal disease and a patient is increasingly likely to develop it the longer he has diabetes. Initially it is often intermittent and can be induced by exercise. Later it becomes continuous and may increase in amount to produce the nephrotic syndrome. As the disease progresses GFR falls and hypertension develops. Diabetic retinopathy usually precedes proteinuria and is aggravated by hypertension. Often there is other evidence of diabetic complications such as neuropathies and vascular disease adding to the patient's misery and rendering management more difficult. Once proteinuria has developed most patients will be in terminal renal failure within 5–10 years.

Diagnosis

In general there are no difficulties in making the diagnosis in a patient with long-standing diabetes who has appropriate histological changes. Occasionally, however, when there is no antecedent history of diabetes mellitus it may be more difficult since chronic renal failure from any cause is associated with carbohydrate intolerance (see p. 141). While it may be important to exclude obstruction in a patient with diabetes mellitus, intravenous urography should be avoided since this may lead to a deterioration in renal function and for this reason ultrasound examination is preferable.

Management

General principles

(a)   ensure the best possible diabetic control (even though there is no good evidence that this delays or reverses renal deterioration);
(b)   ensure good blood pressure control—hypertension and diabetes make a bad combination;
(c)   treat the nephrotic syndrome and chronic renal failure in the same manner as in non-diabetic patients, but modify drug therapy where necessary.

Diabetic control

Most patients will be on insulin. This should be continued but the dose may need reducing since insulin is degraded by the kidneys. Similarly the oral agents or their active metabolites are excreted by the kidneys so that the dose may need modifying. Biguanides which may cause fatal lactic acidosis should be avoided.

Proteinuria

Asymptomatic proteinuria requires an increase in dietary protein. Where the nephrotic syndrome develops, sodium restriction and diuretic therapy will be needed. Where renal failure becomes superimposed on the nephrotic syndrome, protein restriction should be imposed when gastrointestinal symptoms develop, or the blood urea exceeds $55 \, \text{mmol} \, l^{-1}$. However, additional dietary protein should be given if there is significant proteinuria. Conventional carbohydrate restriction will be necessary.

Hypertension

Beta-blockers should be used with caution in those receiving insulin since they may delay recovery from a hypoglycaemic episode. Selective β-blockers such as atenolol or metoprolol are preferable. Diazoxide is best avoided since its capacity to produce hyperglycaemia may make diabetic control more difficult. Other hypotensive agents cause few problems.

By the time a diabetic develops terminal renal failure he usually has evidence of widespread diabetic complications such as retinopathy, cardiovascular disease and autonomic neuropathy. These patients do badly on maintenance dialysis or if they receive a transplant. It may be that continuous ambulatory peritoneal dialysis (CAPD) will prove the most satisfactory alternative.

Diabetes and urinary tract infections and papillary necrosis

Urinary infections are common in diabetics. The following factors may predispose to them:

(a) glycosuria is a good culture medium;

(b)   neuropathic bladder may be present;
(c)   immunity may be impaired.
     Ischaemia of the renal medulla may contribute to the develop-
ment of papillary necrosis, particularly where recurrent infections
occur.

AMYLOIDOSIS

Occurs as:
1   primary condition;
2   secondary to chronic suppurative conditions (rheumatoid arthritis (RA) common);
3   in association with malignancies:
    (a)   multiple myeloma;
    (b)   medullary carcinoma of the thyroid;
    (c)   islet cell tumours of the pancreas;
4   In association with hereditary disorders:
    (a)   deafness, urticaria and amyloidosis;
    (b)   hereditary perireticular amyloidosis;
    (c)   hereditary neuropathic amyloidosis;
    (d)   familial Mediterranean fever.

Pathogenesis

Lesions result from the deposition of protein fibrils composed of
polypeptide chains in the vascular tissues. The amyloid substance
may be one of two types:
1   insoluble product known as AL amyloid which is derived from
a segment of the kappa or (more commonly) the lambda chain of an
immunoglobulin and multiple myeloma.
2   an insoluble protein of nearly constant composition known as
AA amyloid. It is seen more commonly in secondary amyloidosis
and is derived from a serum protein SAA. Either form may be found
in primary amyloidosis.

Pathological lesion

Microscopically, the first renal abnormality consists of hyaline widening of the intercapillary and mesangial regions, with some thick-

ening of the capillary basement membrane. As it progresses the amount of amyloid tissue deposit increases as does the capillary wall thickening, leading to a reduction in the lumen of the capillary. The tubules become atrophic. The main diagnostic feature is the presence of birefringence when the section has been stained with congo red and is viewed in polarized light. Under the electron-microscope amyloid fibrils are apparent, lying against the basement membrane usually between the endothelium and the basement membrane of the glomerulus.

Clinical features

In addition to renal involvement, the heart may be affected leading to heart failure, the nerves may be involved leading to a peripheral neuropathy and there may be deposition in the liver, spleen and lymph nodes so that they become enlarged.

Renal involvement reveals itself clinically as proteinuria which is initially asymptomatic. Later if severe enough, it can cause the nephrotic syndrome and ultimately renal failure. Renal vein thrombosis may complicate renal amyloidosis at which point there is a sudden worsening of the proteinuria with haematuria. Hypertension occurs in about 50% of cases.

Investigations

1 *MSU*: microscopic haematuria, granular and fatty casts, heavy proteinuria.
2 *Biochemistry*: non-specific with decrease in serum albumin if nephrotic and elevation of blood urea and creatinine if in renal failure.
3 *24-hour urine*: 1–20 g proteinuria which is non-selective.
4 *IVU*: renal outlines smooth, size may be increased in early stages but later is often reduced.
5 *Biopsy*: rectal biopsy positive for amyloidosis in 85%, renal biopsy positive in more than 90%.

Management

(a) Symptomatic

Proteinuria requires an adequate protein intake. Once the nephrotic syndrome develops, sodium restriction and diuretic therapy will be needed in addition to the high protein intake (see Chapter 9, p. 74). As renal impairment ensues protein restriction will become necessary.

(b)   Specific

(i)   Where amyloidosis is secondary to a chronic suppurative condition, removal of this focus where possible may halt renal deterioration and may even lead to its reversal. Similarly there may be regression following the treatment of multiple myeloma with the appropriate chemotherapy (corticosteroids and melphalan).
(ii)   Various cytotoxics including chlorambucil, mephalan and azathioprine have been tried but their efficacy remains uncertain.
(iii)   Dimethylsulphoxide (D M S O) has been shown to reduce serum S A A levels and in some cases to improve renal function, although it has not been used in a controlled trial.

In general, patients with amyloidosis do not do as well on maintenance haemodialysis or following transplantation as patients with non-systemic disease.

GOUT

Pathophysiology

Uric acid is the end-product of purine metabolism. It is excreted in the glomerular filtrate, reabsorbed in the proximal tubule and excreted distal to the site of reabsorption. In the majority of patients with a primary abnormality of urate metabolism, no specific defect has been demonstrated.

Raised serum uric acid concentration may occur in patients with malignant disease (particularly myeloproliferative disorders), especially when treated with cytotoxic chemotherapy.

A reduced G F R in patients with renal impairment also leads to increased plasma uric acid levels.

Clinical gout may be associated with the following forms of renal disease:
(a)   chronic gouty nephropathy;
(b)   acute gouty nephropathy;
(c)   urolithiasis.

(a)   Chronic gouty nephropathy

In patients with gout this is the second most common complication after arthritis. It is rare under the age of 40 but increases thereafter and is the most common cause of death in these patients. However it does not seem to reduce their life expectancy by much, if at all. Patients present with nocturia resulting from renal tubular impairment. As the disease progresses hypertension often supervenes and, if urate stones form, loin pain and haematuria may occur.

HISTOLOGY

Chronic gouty nephropathy is characterized by the presence of crystals of uric acid in the tubules and interstitium which provoke a giant cell reaction leading to an interstitial nephropathy (see p. 91).

Investigations

MSU: red cells if calculi present, proteinuria. Plasma uric acid elevated out of proportion to GFR. 24-hour protein excretion 0.5–1 g.
IVU—may demonstrate radiolucent stones.

Management

Symptomatic

It is necessary to control hypertension and urinary infections.

Specific

Give allopurinol, a xanthine oxidase inhibitor. This prevents the conversion of xanthine to uric acid. Although xanthine is relatively insoluble, xanthine stones are not a problem. Allopurinol is well tolerated but it should be given with care to patients with renal impairment. It may cause a vasculitis which requires immediate termination of therapy.

(b)   Acute gouty nephropathy

This is a potential problem in patients with malignant disease, especially myeloproliferative disorders. The massive cellular death which may result from cytotoxic therapy leads to an increase in purine metabolism and uric acid production. This may be precipitated in the tubules, collecting ducts and even in the pelvis and ureters especially if the urine is acid. Clinically the patients present with an acute onset of oliguria or anuria shortly after starting chemotherapy.

Investigations

Urine: red cells and urate crystals
Blood: raised plasma uric acid
IVU, ultrasound or CT scan may show obstruction

Treatment

Alkalinize the urine with oral $NaHCO_3$ or Shohl's solution. Give allopurinol.

In situations where acute gouty nephropathy is likely, prevention is better than cure—give allopurinol prophylactically.

Catheterization of ureters may be necessary followed by alkaline washouts.

Nephrolithiasis

This occurs in 10-25% of patients with gout. The stones are radiolucent and will require the injection of contrast in order to demonstrate them. The clinical features are no different from those seen in other forms of stone disease (see p. 120). Treatment is with allopurinol and, if necessary, surgery.

MULTIPLE MYELOMA

Pathophysiology

Multiple myeloma results from the proliferation of a clone of plasma cells in the bone marrow, causing an overproduction of a particular immunoglobulin or its fragments (heavy or light chains). This 'monoclonal gammopathy' is characterized by the demonstration of a monoclonal band on plasma protein electrophoresis and depression of the other immunoglobulins. In some cases kappa or lambda light chains can be found in the urine in the absence of a 'band' in the plasma. IgG myeloma occurs most commonly (75%) followed by IgA (20%).

Light chain fragments are filtered by glomerular capillaries and are reabsorbed by and catabolized in proximal tubular cells.

Pathological lesions

The kidney may be involved in several different ways.

1 *Myeloma kidney:* this results from the precipitation within the distal tubules of dense eosinophilic hard glassy casts which contain kapppa or lambda chains. These casts may be associated with varying degrees of giant cell reaction. Calcification within casts occurs and tubular atrophy is frequent.

2 Hypercalcaemia: this may result in precipitation of calcium in the tubular epithelium.

3 Amyloidosis: this may be deposited in the kidney in 10% of cases.

4 Infiltration of the kidney by plasma cells occurs rarely.

5 Uric acid deposition.

Clinical features

Patients may present with any combination of the following:

(a) lethargy, malaise;

(b) anaemia;

(c) polyuria and polydipsia secondary to hypercalcaemia;

(d) bone pain resulting from local destruction of bone by plasma cells;

(e) renal involvement

   (i) progressive renal failure—common with light chain and IgD myeloma;

   (ii) nephrotic syndrome due to amyloidosis;

   (iii) Fanconi-like syndrome;

   (iv) urinary tract infections.

Investigations

Blood. Full blood count—anaemia and raised ESR. Reversed albumin/globulin ratio is common. Blood urea and creatinine are elevated where there is renal impairment. Monoclonal gammopathy may be demonstrated by protein electrophoresis.

Urine.   Proteinuria is common and may be shown to be Bence Jones protein.

Bone Marrow.   An increase in plasma cells would be diagnostic of myeloma.

Radiology.   IVU should only be performed with caution since dehydration may lead to the precipitation of protein within the kidney tubules.

Management

The survival in multiple myeloma is inversely related to both the degree of anaemia and renal failure. Where the latter is the result of a myeloma, treatment with cytotoxic agents does not seem to improve the renal function, unless amyloidosis is also present. The patients should be kept well hydrated and in light chain disease it is important to alkalinize the urine. Hypercalcaemia should be vigorously controlled with a high fluid intake and corticosteroids. Hyperuricaemia should be treated with Allopurinol.

SICKLE-CELL ANAEMIA

This is an inherited disorder in which the haemoglobin structure is abnormal so that under conditions of hypoxia, acidosis and hyperosmolarity (such as occurs in the renal medulla) the physicochemical state of the haemoglobin changes so that the cells leak haemoglobin, haemolyse, and become sickle shaped leading to aggregates.

Pathological lesion

Macroscopically, the kidneys are of near normal size. Early on there may be no gross abnormality, but later fine scars are present, presumably as the result of small infarcts.

Microscopically, the glomeruli, especially in the juxtamedullary region, appear prominent because of distension with blood. The afferent and efferent arterioles and vasa recta are engorged with sickle-cells and in the medulla there is oedema, focal scarring and interstitial fibrosis. Papillary necrosis is common.

Clinical features

Patients with the homozygous form are anaemic and suffer 'crises' in which the sickle-cells aggregate and produce small infarcts causing pain in the bones, joints, muscle, abdomen, etc. Haemolysis also occurs causing a worsening of the anaemia. Renal involvement is almost invariable but takes longer to develop in those with the heterozygous form of the disease. It manifests itself clinically by episodes of recurrent haematuria which may be so severe as to warrant nephrectomy. Because of medullary damage and papillary necrosis patients can be shown to have defective tubular function with an inability to concentrate and acidify their urine. There is also an increased incidence of pyelonephritis. Significant proteinuria occurs in 30% and in a much smaller percentage the nephrotic syndrome develops.

Management

It is not possible to correct the underlying abnormality. The attacks of haematuria may settle spontaneously but several treatments, including counteracting medullary hypertonicity and acidity with diuretics, alkalis and hypotonic infusions have been used. Epsilon aminocaproic acid (EACA) has also been used to stem the bleeding. There is experimental evidence that ethacrynic acid may inhibit the tendency to sickle, thus preventing 'crises'.

HAEMOLYTIC URAEMIC SYNDROME AND THROMBOTIC THROMBOCYTOPENIC PURPURA (TTP)

These rare conditions have much in common, both in their pathological appearance and clinical presentation, so that it is easiest to consider them together.

Pathogenesis

The precise pathogenesis is uncertain but it is probable that platelets stick to damaged cell walls causing destruction of erythrocytes as they pass through the affected vessels.

Pathological lesions

Amorphous eosinophilic thrombi which stain with PAS can be demonstrated in the terminal arterioles of many organs; they are probably more extensive in TTP. These thrombi are present in the kidney and may be associated with thickening of the glomular capillary walls progressing to a proliferative picture with crescents.

Clinical features

The patient presents with an acute illness with fever, anaemia, purpura and mild jaundice. Oliguria or anuria supervenes and there may be neurological symptoms with coma, convulsions, paresis and aphasia, particularly in TTP. Table 12.1 shows a comparison of the two conditions.

Table 12.1 Comparison of haemolytic uraemic syndrome and thrombotic thrombocytopenia.

	Haemolytic uraemic syndrome	Thrombotic thrombocytopenia
Age	90% < 4 years but occurs in adults	Max. incidence 10–40 years
Sex	M = F	F > M
Preceding illness	Common; occurs after gastroenteritis, URTI immunization. ? viral related	No preceding illness
Occurs in epidemics	Yes	No
Familial incidence	Yes	Yes
Associated conditions	None	Pregnancy, post-partum 'Pill'
Overall mortality	5–20%	75% within 3 months from neurological damage or haemorrhage

Investigations

The peripheral blood picture shows an anaemia with a thrombocytopenia and often a leucocytosis. A proportion of the erythrocytes are grossly fragmented. There is evidence of haemolysis with a raised reticulocyte count, absent haptoglobins and the presence of methaemalbumin in the plasma. Tests for erythrocyte antibodies are negative. The blood urea and creatinine are raised and the urine contains protein and red cells.

Although recovery may occur, renal impairment may persist and hypertension develops. In some cases anuria persists and cortical necrosis develops, leading to an appearance of tramline calcification on abdominal X-rays.

Treatment

The outcome is varied and the incidence low so that there have been no opportunities to conduct controlled studies of therapeutic agents. Corticosteroids, heparin, warfarin, streptokinase, platelet anti-aggregating agents, such as dipyridamole and cytotoxic agents, and plasma infusions have all been used with varying degrees of success.

LIVER DISEASES

Patients suffering from various liver disorders frequently have renal abnormalities. In addition, extraneous poisons, e.g. carbon tetrachloride (CCl_4), and infections, e.g. Weil's disease, may affect both organs simultaneously.

Obstructive jaundice

These patients' kidneys are particularly vulnerable if they have to undergo surgery. It used to be thought that the renal tubular cells were particularly prone to ischaemic damage if jaundice was present. It is now known that cortical blood flow is reduced probably by a locally active pressor agent, e.g. angiotensin, and the i.v. injection of mannitol during the operation will protect the kidneys.

Chronic active hepatitis and primary biliary cirrhosis

Tubular defects with an inability to excrete acid have been found in chronic hepatidides—these are expressed as hyperchloraemic acidosis and hypokalaemia.

Viral hepatitis

An immune type of glomerulonephritis is associated with acute hepatitis B infections. Chronic hepatitis B carriers can develop membranous glomerular changes and the nephrotic syndrome has been described. 25–40% of patients with polyarteritis nodosa are hepatitis B surface antigen carriers and have evidence of glomerulonephritis.

Glomerular changes in cirrhosis

Glomerular lesions have been known for a long time to occur in cirrhotic patients. Mesangial deposition of IgA is the most consistent finding and may be associated clinically with proteinuria and haematuria.

Renal dysfunction and cirrhosis (hepato-renal syndrome)

In the early stages there is a failure to excrete a salt and water load with a reversal of diurnal rhythm.

Later, these changes become more marked and renal cortical blood flow diminishes. Fluid retention becomes severe with massive ascites and biochemical evidence of renal impairment develops. Worsening of renal function sometimes occurs without any obvious precipitating factor, but usually it follows such an event as a gastrointestinal haemorrhage, septicaemia or paracentesis abdominis.

Blood pressure is low and urine volume is reduced although it is often hypertonic. Total sodium excretion is very low ($< 10 \, \text{mmol/l}$) because hyperaldosteronism causes intense sodium retention. Even so plasma sodium levels are low due to water retention. The failing liver probably loses its ability to metabolize aldosterone, ADH and probably natriuretic hormone.

A low plasma albumin leads to a very low oncotic pressure and the ascites that accompanies it may well have a compressive effect on the renal veins, for drainage of the ascites has a marked effect on renal blood flow.

The renal failure associated with liver cirrhosis has been termed the hepato-renal syndrome, the exact pathophysiological mechanisms of which are ill understood.

Management

The management of the renal problem is of secondary importance to that of dealing with the liver failure. The most important question to be answered is 'Is this patient's total body sodium increased or decreased?' If it is decreased (which is extremely unlikely) then hypovolaemia may be responsible for the reduced urine output and i.v. saline will correct the situation. If, however, there is oedema or ascites then total body sodium must be increased and sodium restriction is *de rigeur*. Remember, a low plasma sodium does not reveal the body sodium content but merely indicates the ratio of sodium to water in the plasma. In the presence of an increased total body sodium, sodium restriction must be instituted and if the plasma sodium drops then the water intake must be cut back to about 500 ml per day. Sodium excretion can be increased by diuretic therapy initially in the form of spironolactone in increasing dosage till the reduction in body weight is of the order of 400 g per day. If, despite using the maximum dose, a naturesis does not occur, a loop diuretic should be added.

When renal failure complicates cirrhosis the patients usually have ascites, jaundice and portal systemic encephalopathy. The urine volume is reduced and in the early stages it may be concentrated; the sodium content is usually below $10 \, mmol \, l^{-1}$. As the condition progresses, the urine may become diluted; the development of severe renal failure usually heralds total body failure and the patient often dies before the plasma creatinine becomes markedly elevated. The mechanism is thought to be that of a disturbed renal circulation with reduction in the cortical flow, together with generalized vasodilation and shunting from various organs including the kidneys. Occasionally, however, a gastrointestinal bleed may precipitate oliguria by being responsible for hypovolaemia.

Do not assume that a reduced urine volume necessarily means renal failure, for the G F R measured by creatinine clearance may be normal—where there is evidence of renal failure consider hypovolaemia. If this is present, give i.v. fluids in the form of salt-poor albumin if the plasma albumin is low. Unless you have cast iron evidence of sodium depletion (no ascites, or oedema and postural hypotension) do not give sodium **in any form**. Treat any other causes of renal failure (nephrotoxins including drugs, obstruction, infection, etc.) Where there is no obvious explanation keep the patient electrolytically and metabolically as stable as possible. If necessary consider dialysis—it is unlikely to alter a rotten prognosis, but is a means of keeping a patient going until spontaneous recovery occurs.

POTASSIUM DEPLETION

CAUSES

1 The commonest source of potassium loss is the intestinal tract. Some is lost by vomiting and renal losses can be enhanced if the vomiting is severe enough to result in metabolic alkalosis. Intestinal malabsorption, ulcerative colitis and purgative abuse all lead to significant potassium losses.

2 Diuretic treatment without potassium supplements.

3 Primary hyperaldosteronism (Conn's syndrome).

4 Cushing's syndrome (corticosteroid treatment).

5 Renal tubular acidosis.

6 Diabetes mellitus.

Pathogenesis

Potassium depletion produces structural changes in both proximal and distal renal tubules—the cells becoming vacuolated. Infection is a common accompaniment.

Clinical features

Impaired urinary concentrating ability leads to polyuria and polydipsia. This functional abnormality is usually reversible although it may take several weeks or months to do so. Irreversible changes, however, have been described.

Treatment

Is that of the underlying condition along with potassium replacement.

PSYCHOGENIC POLYDIPSIA

Occurs in those who are usually mentally disturbed. Females are affected more often than males. The patient presents with polyuria and polydipsia which is indistinguishable from diabetes insipidus. Differentiation can be made by a water deprivation test (without giving the patient prior warning since she is likely to stock up in anticipation). However if the polydipsia has been severe or of long standing, the patient may not be able to concentrate the urine. This is because the urea will have been washed out of the medulla to such an extent that the fluid in the collecting ducts is no longer exposed to a high osmotic force.

RENAL CALCULI

There are several abnormalities which predispose to urinary stone formation and often more than one is present. The following factors may be relevant.
1 Urine supersaturated with a solute.
2 Persistent abnormality of urinary pH so that solubility of a solute is reduced.
3 Renal abnormality which leads to stasis thus allowing stone formation in the stagnant urine.
4 Reduction in inhibitors which help to prevent crystal formation in supersaturated urine.

Renal calculi affect 1-5% of the population—they rarely lead to renal failure and death, but are a major source of misery. The problems that they cause will depend upon their size and the rate at which they develop. They may be found incidentally or they may be responsible for:
(a) ureteric colic—this occurs with the passage of a stone down the ureter into the bladder. The patient suffers from extreme pain which renders him pale, sweaty and even in tears. The pain starts in the loin and radiates down to the groin and testicle in the male or labia in the female;
(b) dull loin ache—this may occur where there is a stone moving around the renal pelvis or causing some degree of obstruction to the one of the calyces or the pelvi-ureteric junction.
(c) association with intractable urinary tract infection.

General principles of management

1   The diagnosis is made from the history and investigations
(a)   examination of the urine for cells ± infection;
(b)   IVU for stones.
2   Consider if surgical intervention is necessary because of persistence of obstruction (usually pelvi-ureteric junction, opposite the body of L2 and at the lower end of the ureter especially if the stone has infection behind it). The position and size of the stones will determine the surgical approach. Large ones, especially in the upper tract, will need an open operation, smaller ones stuck on the lower ureter can often be removed by a Dormier basket. Most small ones (< 1 cm) will pass spontaneously.
3   If possible, determine the chemical mature of the stone by analysis.
4   Look for a metabolic abnormality which may be responsible for them.
5   Assess whether the stones are metabolically active, i.e. whether they are increasing in size and/or number by performing serial abdominal X-rays.
6   Try and slow the rate of stone formation and growth by a high fluid intake (enough to ensure a 24-hour urinary output of three litres including drinking at night) and by correcting metabolic abnormality if present.
   The following metabolic disorders may be associated with renal calculi.

Renal tubular acidosis Type I (distal tubular defect)

The exact cause of stones in this condition is not certain but several factors may contribute:
(a)   high pH decreases the solubility of calcium phosphate;
(b)   some patients have hypercalciuria;
(c)   recurrent infections;
(d)   low urinary citrate.
   These patients present in childhood with stones or nephrocalcinosis (calcification outside the collecting system).

SPECIFIC TREATMENT

Consists in correcting the acidosis with bicarbonate or citrate salts.

Cystinuria

This condition is inherited as an autosomal recessive gene. There is failure of tubular reabsorption of cystine together with lysine, ornithine and arginine. The maximum incidence occurs in the second decade, but can occur at any age. The stones, which are moderately radiopaque, do not occur in everyone with cystinuria (reason unknown).

The diagnosis is made by examination of stones, by demonstrating cystine crystals in urine (hexagonal) or a raised cystine excretion by the nitroprusside test. Chromatography of the urine will demonstrate the excess of amino acids present.

TREATMENT

1   Alkalinize the urine.
2   Ensure daily urine volumes of 3–4 litres.
3   Low methionine-containing diet may help.
4   Penicillamine if all else fails.

Hyperoxaluria

Primary hyperoxaluria is inherited as an autosomal recessive. It is the most malignant of all the stone diseases since it leads to calcium oxalate deposition in the kidneys and urinary tract, the blood vessels, the myocardium and joints, and usually leads to death. Renal stones and nephrocalcinosis lead to progressive renal failure and cardiac deposits lead to conduction problems. 80% of patients are in terminal renal failure by the age of 20 years.

The diagnosis is made by measuring urinary oxalate excretion. The analysis of stones is unhelpful because many mixed stones contain oxalate. Treatment is generally unsatisfactory, though oxalate production rate can sometimes be modified by pyridoxine and orthophosphates. Dialysis treatment rarely prevents the cardiac manifestations of the disease.

Secondary oxaluria can occur:
(a)   after ethylene glycol intoxication;
(b)   after a methoxyflurane anaesthesia;
(c)   after jejuno-ileal bypass surgery;
(d)   in inflammatory bowel disease.

Urinary stones and renal failure can occur in some instances, and treatment is usually unsatisfactory.

Xanthinuria

Occurs as a rare autosomal recessive disorder where there is a deficiency of xanthine oxidase so that there is increased urinary xanthine excretion and a reduced plasma and urinary acid concentration. A third of the patients develop calculi which are characteristically radiolucent. Treatment consists of alkalinizing the urine to increase solubility.

Hypercalcaemia and hypercalciuria

CAUSES OF HYPERCALCAEMIA

1 Primary hyperparathyroidism.
2 Sarcoidosis.
3 Vitamin D intoxication.
4 Associated with malignancy
   (a) bony metastases;
   (b) PTH secreting tumour;
   (c) related to prostaglandins.
5 Multiple myeloma.
6 Others
   (a) hyperthyroidism;
   (b) Addisons disease;
   (c) mild alkali syndrome;
   (d) immobilization following fractures or inpatients with Paget's disease.

CAUSES OF HYPERCALCIURIA

(i) Hypercalcaemia may be associated with hypercalciuria and stone formation. Its treatment is that of the underlying condition.
(ii) Idiopathic hypercalciuria is probably a mixture of conditions—often the mechanism is ill understood. Certainly one group (predominantly males) have high intestinal calcium absorption. The serum calcium is normal, but the phosphate may be low and there is hypercalciuria. It looks as though the defect in these patients may be an increase in plasma $1,25(OH)_2D_3$, perhaps stimulated by the low

plasma phosphate. The hallmark of the condition is an increased 24-hour urinary calcium excretion which returns to normal if the patient is fasted. This distinguishes it from the form in which a renal leak is the main problem (see below). The stones are a mixture of oxalate and phosphate and are radiopaque. Treatment consists of reducing dietary calcium (less milk and cheese) and reducing intestinal calcium absorption with calcium-binding agents (cellulose phosphate). Oral phosphate has been advocated on the grounds that it increases urinary pyrophosphate which helps to prevent crystal formation. However it may be that by increasing plasma phosphate it leads to a reduced $1,25(OH)_2D_3$ level.

The second group are those with a renal leak of calcium and in whom the urinary calcium excretion remains high, even when the dietary intake is reduced. Treatment by reducing calcium intake will not help, therefore, and may even be deleterious, since the calcium lost will come from bone, leading to osteoporosis. In this condition a thiazide diuretic is indicated since it will reduce urinary calcium excretion (a loop diuretic like frusemide has the opposite effect). Stones in this group seem to start as urate crystals so that allopurinol has been used to prevent the initiation of the crystal.

It is thought that a lack of crystal inhibitors, such as acid micropolysaccharides, and possibly an increase in urate or oxalate excretion are the main factors here. A high fluid intake together with allopurinol, thiazides and oral phosphates have been used but their efficiency is uncertain.

Finally, there is a big group (25-50%) in whom the urinary calcium excretion is normal.

Hyperuricaemia (see p. 110)

Treatment with allopurinol.

Gut disease

There is an increased incidence of renal calculi in those with a shortened bowel (resulting from surgical resection, bypass operations or because of fistula formation). The stones are composed either of urates (resulting from altered urinary pH) or oxalates. Oxalate stones are thought to occur because increased faecal fats bind calcium so that it is not available to form insoluble calcium oxalate within the gut lumen. Intestinal absorption of oxalate and its urinary excretion are therefore increased.

Finally it is worth putting things into perspective. Only 1% of those with calculi will have an inherited tubular or enzymatic disorder, while hyperuricaemia will be responsible for 5–40% and primary hyperparathyroidism for 5%. The remainder will belong to the group which includes idiopathic hypercalciuria and probable inhibitor deficiency. Thus, although a student is likely to know that stones occur in cystinuria, he is unlikely ever to see a case.

Chapter 13
Chronic Renal Failure

The progression of diffuse renal disease can lead to chronic renal failure which if untreated will inevitably lead to death.

Causes of chronic renal failure

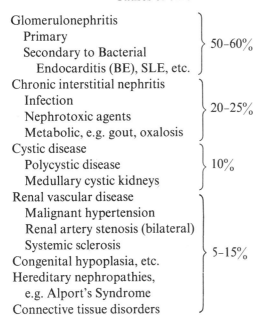

Glomerulonephritis
   Primary
   Secondary to Bacterial
      Endocarditis (BE), SLE, etc. } 50–60%

Chronic interstitial nephritis
   Infection
   Nephrotoxic agents
   Metabolic, e.g. gout, oxalosis } 20–25%

Cystic disease
   Polycystic disease
   Medullary cystic kidneys } 10%

Renal vascular disease
   Malignant hypertension
   Renal artery stenosis (bilateral)
   Systemic sclerosis
Congenital hypoplasia, etc.
Hereditary nephropathies,
   e.g. Alport's Syndrome
Connective tissue disorders } 5–15%

Stages

1 Diminished renal reserve.
Asymptomatic patient with normal blood urea but diminished GFR. Stressful complications such as infection, bleeding or dehydration will cause blood urea to rise but the patient suffers no systemic upset. Biochemical results return to normal eventually.

2 Impaired renal function.

Patient asymptomatic but with abnormally high blood urea and creatinine levels even under normal conditions. These worsen and may be accompanied by symptoms under conditions of stress but may return to previous levels when the stressful situation is relieved. This condition is sometimes called 'acute on chronic' renal failure.

3 Decompensated renal failure or uraemia.

At this stage the blood urea and creatinine levels are permanently raised to such a level that the patient is symptomatic.

Caution

The cause of renal failure should as far as possible be established for the simple reason that some conditions may, if corrected, result in partial or full functional recovery.

Potentially reversible causes

Urinary tract obstruction
Urinary tract infection
Hypertensive renal disease
Bacterial endocarditis or shunt nephritis
Hypokalaemic nephropathy
Hypercalcaemia
Hyperuricaemia
Nephrotoxic nephropathy, e.g. analgesics
Connective tissue disorders

Possible clues may be obtained from careful history taking and clinical examination.

A history of long-standing urinary symptoms, nocturia or chronic ill health would indicate chronic renal failure, and if on examination, anaemia, pigmentation, hypertension, pericarditis and evidence of renal osteodystrophy were found, the chances of irreversible renal disease would be high. If, in addition, radiological examination of the kidneys showed them to be shrunken or grossly scarred, the diagnosis of chronic renal failure would be well established.

On the contrary, if the duration of illness were short, and the kidneys were found to be of normal size radiologically, the possibility of a reversible process would be worth exploring; therefore, further investigations should be undertaken, with the hope of finding obstruction, infection, electrolyte abnormalities or nephrotoxic drug ingestion which may be reversible.

Pathology

1 Diseases of the renal glomeruli (see Chapter 8) are by far the commonest causes of chronic renal failure. The natural history of the condition will depend upon:

(a) the amount and the nature of the initial damage inflicted;

(b) the ability of the host to repair the damage;

(c) the eradication of the insulting agent.

Ironically tissue repair leading to fibrosis can result in hypertension which, if untreated, may cause further progressive vascular damage to the kidneys.

2 Whereas glomerulonephritis will attack normal healthy kidneys, other disease processes leading to chronic renal failure are more often likely to affect congenitally abnormal tissues, e.g. dysplastic kidneys, cystic kidneys, malpositioned (or ectopic) kidneys and ureters. Acquired abnormalities, e.g. obstruction, stones or neuropathic conditions of the bladder may be preventable, but if untreated will certainly lead to destruction. The common denominator of all these anomalies is urinary infection which may or may not be symptomatic.

3 Recurrent damage resulting in interstitial fibrosis can be inflicted by:

(a) repeated urinary infections in infants with vesico-ureteric reflux. Scarring and stunting or renal growth results;

(b) long-term ingestion of analgesic compounds (containing aspirin and phenacetin). Renal papillary necrosis is a common complication and calcification of the papillae can be seen on X-ray. Infection and/or ureteric obstruction are relatively common.

(c) glomerular damage may be produced by certain drugs such as gold salts, penicillamine, hydralazine, etc. Usually, if the drugs are discontinued as soon as evidence of damage appears, progressive renal destruction can be avoided.

(d) chronic infection by viruses (hepatitis B or measles) or by bacteria (*Staphylococcus albus* in ventriculo-atrial shunt infections) result in chronic immune complex deposition in glomerular basement membranes.

4 Genetic predisposition—many inherited conditions such as polycystic disease, Alport's syndrome, Fabry's disease, oxalosis and gout,
etc., lead to CRF.
5 Hypertension can be the cause or result of renal malfunction.
Effective treatment is mandatory whatever the cause.

The intact nephron hypothesis

Progressive destruction of kidneys could affect all nephrons equally
or in sequence. Histopathology would suggest a patchy destruction,
and microdissection studies have supported this, because, as popula-
tions of nephrons are destroyed, the remaining single nephron GFR's
rise under the stimulus of the solute load. In practice as GFR falls
patients develop polyuria due to an osmotic diuresis.

Mechanisms of uraemia

The syndrome of chronic renal failure has been attributed to the
accumulation of 'uraemic toxins' in the blood as a result of a falling
glomerular filtration rate. Many of these toxins are not identifiable
by ordinary biochemical means. It is generally believed that their
toxic effect is mediated via the various enzymatic processes in the
body. Those affected are lactic dehydrogenase, membrane ATPase,
oxidative phosphorylation, xanthine oxidase and possibly transke-
tolase. Furthermore, electrolyte and water balance is deranged, vitamin D and erythropoietin metabolism impaired, parathyroid function excessively stimulated and renin responses are inappropriate.

Symptoms

There are symptoms which tend to be specific for certain conditions,
e.g. back pain, fever, shivering attacks and dysuria in patients with
recurrent urinary tract infections. Haematuria occurs in polycystic
disease, urinary tract infection, some forms of glomerulonephritis,
carcinoma of the kidneys or urinary tract. However, as renal failure
develops, many non-specific symptoms appear regardless of the
aetiology (see Table 13.1).

Table 13.1 Non-specific symptoms.

Symptoms	Causes
Tiredness, loss of energy	Anaemia
Dyspnoea, orthopnoea	Heart failure
Kussmaul respiration	Acidosis
Oedema	Congestive heart failure (CHF), hypoproteinaemia, overhydration
Headaches, blurred vision, teichopsia	Hypertension
Hiccoughs, nausea, vomiting	Gastritis, peptic ulcer
Diarrhoea	Enterocolitis
Bruising	Qualitative platelet defect
Itching	? Hyperphosphataemia
Chest pain	Pericarditis, ischaemic heart disease (IHD)
Drowsiness, loss of memory, twitching, convulsions, coma	Encephalopathy
Paraesthesiae, numbness, motor weakness	Peripheral neuropathy
Bone pain, fractures, joint swelling	Renal osteodystrophy
Skin pigmentation	Chromogens, melanin

Biochemical abnormalities

Blood

1 PROTEIN METABOLITES

Blood levels of urea, creatinine, uric acid, guanidine and phenolic substances all increase as renal failure develops.

2 HYDROGEN IONS

Failure of tubular function leads to retention of hydrogen ions. Titratable and free acid excretion falls, as well as ammonia production and excretion; furthermore, increased catabolism tends to increase the H^+ load. Patients with tubular abnormalities, e.g. interstitial nephropathies and polycystic disease, tend to become acidotic at an earlier stage of renal impairment than those with glomerulonephritis.

3 POTASSIUM

Normal balance is maintained until renal failure is advanced, but increased catabolism, haemolysis, excessive intake of potassium or K^+-retaining diuretics will increase the plasma levels. However, when GFR falls below 10 ml min^{-1}, potassium retention usually occurs. Hypokalaemia occurs rarely in renal failure and is usually caused by drugs such as diuretics, steroids and outdated tetracyclines which increase urinary K^+ losses.

4 SODIUM

This is not usually altered unless excessive water retention has occurred leading to dilutional hyponatraemia. Hyperlipidaemic states can lead to a falsely low serum sodium. True sodium depletion is rare but is sometimes associated with chronic pyelonephritis.

5 CALCIUM

Intestinal absorption is impaired in chronic renal failure probably due to a defect in vitamin D metabolism. Plasma calcium levels tend to be normal or low and are often associated with increased parathyroid activity.

6 PHOSPHORUS

This is retained when the GFR falls below 30 ml min^{-1}. The reduction in tubular reabsorption of filtered phosphate is under parathyroid hormone (PTH) control and, as phosphate retention occurs, PTH levels tend to rise. Metastatic calcification commonly occurs if the calcium and phosphorus product reaches a high level (>4.4).

7 MAGNESIUM

Magnesium balance is normal in chronic renal failure. This is probably due to the fact that diets tend to have low magnesium contents. Isolated estimation of plasma magnesium levels tend to be high or high normal.

8 GLUCOSE

As a rule this remains normal. However, glucose intolerance does occur in chronic renal failure and a formal glucose tolerance test is usually abnormal. This is probably due to abnormal peripheral metabolism rather than a lack of insulin.

9 PLASMA PROTEINS

These are usually normal unless renal disease has been accompanied by the nephrotic syndrome. As the GFR falls, less protein tends to be lost in the urine so that plasma albumin levels tend to return to normal at very low GFRs.

10 ALKALINE PHOSPHATASE

This enzyme is sometimes an indication of bone turnover, and, in growing children and patients with renal osteodystrophy, high levels can be found.

11 URIC ACID

The level of uric acid remains normal until the creatinine clearance falls below $20\,ml\,min^{-1}$. After that blood levels rise steadily.

It must be remembered that primary hyperuricaemia related to gout may cause chronic interstitial nephropathy, and this should not be confused with secondary hyperuricaemia. Furthermore, elevation of uric acid can occur in myelomatosis, reticulosis (especially during cytotoxic therapy), polycythaemia, and after status epilepticus.

12 HYPERLIPIDAEMIA

Hypertriglyceridaemia is common in chronic renal failure. The aetiology is unknown but may be related to high carbohydrate diets.

Urine

The volume of urine is variable and is not a reliable guide to renal function. Its biochemical composition is important to evaluate.

1 CREATININE CLEARANCE

This is measured by applying the equation UV/P where U is the urine creatinine concentration, V the minute volume and P the plasma creatinine concentration. Creatinine is filtered by the glomeruli and small quantities are excreted by the renal tubules so that the creatinine clearance slightly overestimates glomerular filtration. Furthermore, chromogens can interfere with the estimation if colorimetric methods are used.

2 URINARY PROTEIN

This is of limited diagnostic use in chronic renal disease, however severe proteinuria leading to the nephrotic syndrome ($>5g$ day^{-1}) eventually leads to hypoalbuminaemia. As renal function deteriorates, the amount of protein filtered by the glomeruli tends to fall to approximately $1-2g$ day^{-1} thereby restoring, to some extent, protein balance.

3 URINE CONCENTRATION

It invariably falls so that in chronic renal failure, plasma and urine osmolalities are approximately equal ($280-300$ mmol kg^{-1}) (specific gravity 1010). This is known as isosthenuria, and even after dehydration or vasopressin injections, the concentration remains fixed.

4 URINE ACIDIFICATION

This becomes defective because of the reduced excretion of titratable acid in combination with phosphate and reduced ammonia excretion. Hydrogen ions are therefore retained.

5 URINARY SODIUM LEVELS

These fall as GFR falls. Rarely, in patients with congenital or acquired tubulo-interstitial abnormalities, the loss of ability to reabsorb sodium by the tubules leads to a 'sodium-losing nephritis'.

Clinical problems

Hypertension

Hypertension, which is a common accompaniment of chronic renal failure, has an accelerating effect on the rate of decline in renal function. Though the renin-angiotensin system may well have a part to play in its early development, as renal function dwindles, the influence of salt and water retention becomes overwhelming. Salt restriction and dialysis will control the blood pressure in a few patients but antihypertensive drugs are usually necessary.

A small number of patients with very resistant renin-dependent hypertension may need bilateral nephrectomy.

Heart failure

Fluid retention is not uncommon in oliguric patients who take in excess salt and water. Occasionally heart failure will develop, particularly in those with ischaemic heart disease or uraemic cardiomyopathy.

Treatment is by salt and water restriction, diuretics, vasodilators, and dialysis. As an emergency, venesection could be performed and 200–500 ml of blood removed from an antecubital vein.

Pericarditis

A fibrinous pericarditis may occur in patients with endstage renal failure and may give rise to chest pain which is sometimes aggravated by deep breathing and lying down. Characteristic ECG changes are rare. Treatment with indomethacin or steroids may be useful in alleviating symptoms and diminishing the intensity of the friction rub.

The aetiology of this condition is not known, but it usually disappears when effective dialysis treatment is established. Care must be taken during dialysis because total heparinization can sometimes cause intrapericardial bleeding and cardiac tamponade.

Anaemia

A normochromic normocytic anaemia invariably accompanies chronic renal failure. Examination of a blood film will often show deformed or crenated erythrocytes—these are known as 'burr cells' and are characteristic. Leucocytes and platelets appear normal but platelet aggregation is impaired.

CAUSES OF ANAEMIA

1 Lack of Erythropoietic factor.
2 Haemolysis.
3 Chronic blood loss.
4 Deficiency of haematinics in diet.
5 Bone marrow suppression.

2,3 diphosphoglycerate (DPG)

In chronic renal failure patients adapt fairly well to severe degrees of anaemia. This may in part be due to overproduction of 2,3 diphosphoglycerate (DPG) which has the potential of shifting the oxygen dissociation curve to the right, therefore making oxygen more available to tissues.

Gastrointestinal complications or symptoms

Hiccoughs, nausea, anorexia and vomiting are common, and upper gastrointestinal tract bleeding may occur. 'Uraemic gastritis' is often blamed for these symptoms but no doubt in many cases, they are centrally mediated. Symptoms are often relieved by reducing protein intake, and a fall in blood urea may be observed concomitantly. Antiemetic drugs such as metoclopramide or chlorpromazine may sometimes be necessary.

Intractable diarrhoea may occur as the result of an enterocolitis. Exclusion of other lower bowel pathology by sigmoidoscopy and barium enema is obligatory before symptomatic treatment is given.

Treatment by dialysis improves gastrointestinal symptoms rapidly and the well maintained dialysis patient should be able to enjoy a reasonably liberal diet without fear of symptoms.

Renal osteodystrophy

Renal osteodystrophy (see p. 137) is the term given to the bony abnormality which occurs in patients with chronic renal failure.

Histologically there are changes of either osteomalacia (or rickets if the epiphyses have not fused) or hyperparathyroidism which occur either singularly or in combination. In addition osteosclerosis (increased bone mass) may occur initially but with increasing duration of dialysis this gives way to osteoporosis. The pathophysiology is complex and incompletely understood.

Neurological

Peripheral neuropathy

Recognized since the advent of dialysis as patients now live long enough to manifest this condition. (Exclude diabetes mellitus, amyloid and collagen disorders.)

The cause is unknown—possibly a dialysable toxin. Dialysis may aggravate condition at first, but if dialysis efficiency is improved, condition may regress. Transplantation is curative unless nerves are completely destroyed.

CHARACTERISTICS

Peripheral, mixed sensory/motor neuropathy
Initial symptoms—numbness, paraesthesiae, restlessness in legs (Ekbom's syndrome)
First signs—depressed ankle jerks, loss of vibration sense
Later weakness and hypoaesthesiae. Loss of ankle and knee jerks
Drop foot
Upper limbs may be affected but much less common

Treatment is by dialysis at earliest possible opportunity.

Encephalopathy

CHARACTERISTICS

Intellectual deterioration, forgetfulness, depression
Drowsiness
Myoclonus, tremors (asterixis)
Elileptiform convulsions
Coma

All these symptoms are probably due to the accumulation of metabolic toxins and are reversible by dialysis. Occasionally water intoxication and electrolyte abnormalities may contribute. Overvigorous haemodialysis can aggravate the condition initially, for differences between intra- and extracellular osmotic pressures and bicarbonate levels may lead to cerebral oedema and depression of the respiratory centre. This state of disequilibrium can be improved by hypertonic infusions of dextrose but is best avoided by a gentler introduction to dialysis.

Management of CRF

Long-term management depends upon whether patients are considered suitable for dialysis and transplantation later. If long-term treatment is not contemplated, all efforts should be made to alleviate symptoms and to slow down the rate of decline in renal failure.

Diet It has been traditional to restrict dietary protein intake to approximately 0.25–0.5 g/kg/day in order to allay the gastrointestinal symptoms associated with advancing uraemia. However, there is some evidence that earlier protein restriction might be beneficial in slowing the deterioration in GFR. Proteins containing high proportions of essential amino acids (e.g. meat and eggs) are most efficiently metabolized in the body in the presence of adequate calories (200–3000 kcal) so that some care needs to be taken to ensure the correct proportions of proteins, carbohydrates and fats.

Salt and water Allowances should be according to the patient's ability to excrete them. Hypertensive patients and those with fluid retention must obviously be restricted, whereas those who are capable to excreting salt and water can be allowed extra. Daily weighing and measurement of intake and output should be reasonable guides to replacement.

Potassium Hyperkalaemia rarely develops until the GFR falls below 10 ml min^{-1}. Exceptions to this rule occur if the patient becomes hypercatabolic due to infection or if he has exceeded his normal dietary allowance. Frequent monitoring of plasma potassium should be performed when the GFR falls below 10 ml/min. If these levels exceed 5.5 mmol L^{-1}, dietary restriction should be enforced, and it may be necessary to add exchange resins (calcium resonium) 15 g tds on a regular basis.

Prescribing of drugs (see Chapter 21)

Great care needs to be exercised when prescribing drugs to patients in renal failure. Their route of excretion and toxic side-effects should be known and, if necessary, their doses should be modified and blood levels monitored.

Long-term management (see Chapters 16, 17 and 18)

Any patient considered for long-term dialysis or transplantation should start dialysis treatment before debilitating complications such as pericarditis and peripheral neuropathy develop. It is difficult to set an arbitrary treatment level for blood urea or creatinine clearance, for individual patients vary considerably in their somatic responses to metabolic derangements. Symptoms should always take precedence over biochemical figures, so that an anorectic patient on a 30 g day^{-1} protein diet who has severe hypertension and pericarditis will need urgent dialysis, even though his blood urea is 30 mmol l-1 and creatinine 900 μmol l^{-1}, whereas an asymptomatic patient with a blood urea of 50 mmol l^{-1} and creatinine of 1200 μmol l^{-1} could afford to wait a little longer. The decision finally depends upon available dialysis space, but as a general rule, a blood creatinine level of over 1000 μmol l^{-1} should stimulate one to make dialysis arrangements in the near future.

Metabolic consequences of chronic renal failure

Osteomalacia (rickets)

Bone histology from patients with chronic renal failure shows an increase in unmineralised bone (osteoid) similar to that seen in nutritional osteomalacia. Both conditions are characterized by reduced intestinal calcium absorption but, whereas the administration of physiological amounts of vitamin D to patients with nutritional osteomalacia corrects intestinal malabsorption of calcium and heals the abnormal bone, it has no effect in chronic renal failure. The explanation for this vitamin D resistance in chronic renal failure became apparent when it was appreciated that vitamin D itself was inactive but underwent a series of conversions into metabolically active forms, in much the same way as cholesterol is converted into hormones by the adrenal cortex. The metabolism of vitamin D is shown here.

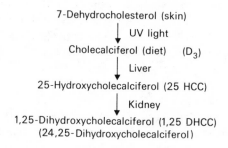

7-Dehydrocholesterol (skin)

↓ UV light

Cholecalciferol (diet)   (D_3)

↓ Liver

25-Hydroxycholecalciferol (25 HCC)

↓ Kidney

1,25-Dihydroxycholecalciferol (1,25 DHCC)
(24,25-Dihydroxycholecalciferol)

1,25-Dihydroxy vitamin D has been shown to be the active component of Vitamin D certainly in terms of stimulating intestinal calcium absorption. The role of 24,25-Dihydroxy vitamin D remains uncertain. Plasma levels of 1,25-Dihydroxy vitamin D are low in patients with chronic renal failure, and oral administration of physiological amounts of this metabolite will overcome intestinal malabsorption of calcium where the parent compound is inactive. However, 1,25-Dihydroxy vitamin D has proved disappointing therapy for the osteomalacic component of renal osteodystrophy (see below).

In addition to abnormalities of vitamin D metabolism itself, there are probably other factors which are pertinent in the aetiology of osteomalacia. Patients with chronic renal failure are likely to be slightly vitamin D deficient since they are often anorexic because of their uraemia and hence have a poor vitamin D intake. Periods of ill health may also result in the patient getting out into the fresh air less often so that there is less chance of ultraviolet light acting upon skin to provide vitamin D. Finally, there is evidence that in some units the aluminium content of the water which is used to make up the dialysate is high and this, in some way, predisposes towards the development of osteomalacia.

Hyperparathyroidism

Hypersecretion of parathyroid hormone takes place in response to hypocalcaemia. This latter occurs for two main reasons:

(a)   intestinal malabsorption of calcium resulting from impaired production of 1,25-Dihydroxy vitamin D as discussed above.

(b)   secondary to phosphate retention. As GFR falls there is a concomitant reduction in phosphate excretion leading to its retention, and consequently an elevated plasma phosphate concentration. This in turn depresses the plasma calcium level thereby stimulating parathyroid gland secretion. Since one of the actions of parathyroid hormone is to increase urinary phosphate excretion the potential biochemical perturbation is prevented. Progressive reduction in GFR will lead to further cycles of changing, each culminating in an increased parathyroid hormone secretion which at very low levels of GFR will be unable to maintain biochemical homeostasis. The term 'tertiary' hyperparathyroidism is said to occur when the parathyroid gland no longer responds appropriately to the plasma calcium level and behaves autonomously.

Osteosclerosis

This probably occurs in response to parathyroid hypersecretion and is of no clinical significance.

Osteoporosis

This probably occurs for a variety of reasons but calcium deficiency is probably the most important.

Clinical features associated with renal osteodystrophy

1   Bone pain, fracture and deformity.

2   Metastatic calcification. This may occur in blood vessels causing difficulty with vascular access and renal transplantation. It is also seen in peri-articular tissue producing joint pain (pseudo gout) and may also be deposited in the eyes giving rise to inflammation.

3   Proximal myopathy leading to difficulty in climbing stairs and getting out of a chair.

4   Pruritus which may in part be related to hyperparathyroidism.

LABORATORY FINDINGS

Biochemical tests are not diagnostic for either osteomalacia or hyperparathyroidism although, in general, the plasma calcium is low in the former and at the upper limit of normal in the latter, except in tertiary hyperparathyroidism where the plasma calcium may be elevated. The alkaline phosphatase is raised when the bone disease is severe. The plasma phosphate is generally elevated and a raised calcium phosphate product is likely to predispose to the development of metastatic calcification. The immunoreactive parathyroid hormone concentration is invariably elevated but correlates poorly with the extent of disease assessed clinically because the assay detects biologically inactive fragments.

X-RAY FINDINGS

Osteomalacia—unlike nutritional osteomalacia Looser's zones are uncommon.

Hyperparathyroidism—subperiosteal erosions of the phalanges and erosion of the outer third of the clavicle, a pepper pot skull, rugger jersey spine and rib fractures are all seen in hyperparathyroidism. X-rays may also show evidence of metastatic calcification in blood vessels, etc.

Treatment

1 Phosphate binding agents are given with meals so that insoluble aluminium phosphate is formed and high phosphate levels prevented.

Aluminium compounds, such as aluminium hydroxide or carbonate are usually used.

2 Hyperparathyroidism if mild and not associated with a raised plasma calcium responds to treatment with 1,25 Dihydroxy vitamin D or its synthetic analogue 1α-Hydroxy-vitamin D in a daily oral dose of $1-2\,\mu g$. However, if the disease is severe, particularly in those with hypercalcaemia, parathyroidectomy is usually necessary.

3 Osteomalacia has in general not proved amenable to treatment with 1,25 Dihydroxy vitamin D. Some other form is usually necessary such as the parent compound in a daily dose of 100 000 units. 25 Hydroxy vitamin D or dihydrotachysterol have been used as alternatives.

Endocrine abnormalities

These are common; their basis is uncertain but some or all of the following facts may be important.
1 There often appears to be end organ resistance. Retained 'middle molecules' may block hormone receptors to produce this effect.
2 Trophic hormone release is often inappropriately low (again possibly due to 'middle molecules' blocking receptors).
3 The kidney is the site of degradation of several hormones and in chronic renal failure this may be impaired leading to an increased hormone half life.
4 Hormones may be displaced from their carrier proteins by 'middle molecules'.

Thyroid disease

Patients with chronic renal failure often have proptosis and exophthalmos yet in other respects appear hypothyroid. They are slow, feel the cold and may have a reduced basal metabolic rate. At first sight thyroid function tests would support the diagnosis of hypothyroidism with the thyroxine (T_4) and triiodothyronine (T_3) at or below the lower limit of normal. However, unlike true hypothyroidism, the plasma thyroid stimulating hormone (TSH) level is not elevated and there is a delayed TSH response to thyrotrophin releasing hormone (TRH) injection with a generally flat curve. Thyroid antibodies are negative. In the majority, supplementation with thyroxine appears to be of no benefit, and should be reserved for the few patients who have an elevated plasma TSH level. Thyroid function remains abnormal when patients receive haemodialysis but returns to normal following successful renal transplantation.

Abnormalities of carbohydrate metabolism

Chronic renal failure is associated with impaired glucose tolerance in that, although the fasting plasma glucose is usually normal, hyperglycaemia often follows a glucose load. This hyperglycaemia is associated with plasma insulin levels which are greater than would be expected, suggesting that there is peripheral insulin resistance. Although elevated levels of both growth hormone and glucagon may be partly responsible for the carbohydrate (CHO) abnormality they are not the whole story; carbohydrate intolerance may improve or even return to normal when the patient starts haemodialysis, yet these hormones remain elevated.

Hyperglycaemia in renal failure is rarely severe enough to warrant treatment, and its main significance lies in the difficulties which it may cause when trying to decide whether a patient has diabetic renal disease or hyperglycaemia occurring in chronic renal failure due to some other condition. The diagnosis of diabetic nephropathy, therefore, must rest on a previous history of carbohydrate intolerance and the characteristic pathological changes. Paradoxically, although hyperglycaemia is common, renal failure may be complicated by hypoglycaemia which may occur either spontaneously or in diabetic patients who have become uraemic, even though there has been no change in their insulin dosage. The kidney is the normal site of insulin degradation and in uraemia there is a prolonged insulin half life, but, in addition to this, impaired glyconeogenesis also seems to occur. In the diabetic, reduction of insulin dosage may be all that is required, but spontaneous hypoglycaemia may be a trap for the unwary. This may occur in a patient undergoing peritoneal dialysis where some of the sugar content of the solution will be absorbed and stimulate insulin secretion. Since the half life of insulin is prolonged, cessation of peritoneal dialysis may be accompanied by hypoglycaemia.

Abnormalities of sexual function

Men

Men with chronic renal failure suffer from decreased libido and potency of varying degrees. On examination there is often testicular atrophy and histology shows decreased spermatogenesis. In these patients the plasma testosterone is reduced and their gonadotrophins, although higher than those seen in normal individuals, are not as high as would be expected for the plasma testosterone levels. There seems to be an inability of the testes to secrete normal amounts of testosterone and there is also a reduced ability of the pituitary to secrete trophic hormones.

In addition the plasma prolactin levels are elevated (see below) and this may be an important factor. However, in addition to the endocrine abnormalities, there are other factors which contribute to impotence such as malaise resulting from uraemia, medication (particularly hypotensive agents), and possibly uraemic neuropathy affecting the automonic nerves. Although haemodialysis does not affect the endocrine abnormalities, sexual performance may improve, probably as a result of the patient's increased sense of well being. Following renal transplantation sexual function returns to normal.

Women

Decreased libido also occurs in women. In those who are premenopausal, amenorrhoea may accompany chronic renal failure, and where menstruation does occur it is often irregular and the cycles are generally anovulatory. The plasma progesterone is usually very low and the oestrogen may also be difficult to detect. However, despite these low levels, the plasma gonadatrophins are low or normal. In patients who are post-menopausal, however, the plasma gonadatrophin levels become grossly elevated, suggesting that in this situation the pituitary is capable of response. On dialysis there is no change in the endocrine levels but women may suffer from menorrhagia, as a result of heparin given during each dialysis treatment. As in men, the plasma prolactin levels are raised and this may be a contributing factor to the decreased sexual function. Although the majority of women have anovulatory cycles, those who do ovulate may become pregnant although it is exceptional for the pregnancy to continue to a successful conclusion. The libido and potency return to normal following successful transplantation, and there are now many children born to mothers who have undergone this operation. Immunosuppression does not appear to result in an increased instance of fetal abnormalities.

The numerous attempts at trying to relieve the sexual disorders in both men and women attest to their inadequacy. Sexual counselling is probably the most significant help which can be offered.

Prolactin

High prolactin levels have been found in both men and women with renal failure. This may well contribute to the decreased potency and has been suggested to be responsible for galactorrhoea in women and gynaecomastia in men. However, this may not prove to be the whole story. Bromocriptine has been given to patients to reduce prolactin levels, but it has been associated with a high incidence of side-effects, notably postural hypotension (although it has, at least in males, improved potency).

Gastrin

Patients with chronic renal failure have a higher incidence of peptic ulceration, and barium meal examination usually reveals increased rugal folds suggesting hyperacidity. High plasma gastrin levels can be shown to occur in this situation but it is not entirely certain whether this is responsible for the high incidence of peptic ulceration.

Chapter 14
Hypertension and the Kidney

Hypertension and renal disease are interrelated; hypertension may lead to renal disease and renal disease itself may result in hypertension.

Causes of hypertension

1 Essential
This is responsible for 95% of all cases of hypertension. Its aetiology is not understood and the diagnosis is made when other secondary causes have been excluded.

2 Renal artery stenosis
This occurs from narrowing due to:
  (a) atheroma;
  (b) fibromuscular hyperplasia. Reduced renal perfusion results in increased renin secretion from the juxtaglomerular cells resulting in an increased production of angiotensin II. Angiotensin II is the most potent physiological vaso-constrictor known and also stimulates the adrenal to produce aldosterone so that there is sodium retention. Clinically the diagnosis is suggested by a renal bruit. An intravenous urogram (I V U) may show the following characteristic features:
    (i) The affected kidney is smaller than the contralateral kidney by 1.5 cm or more.
    (ii) The nephrogram is delayed.
    (iii) The nephrogram, once developed, is more intense than on the contralateral side.
Unfortunately all three features are only present in about 20% of patients with this condition. A Hippuran scan shows a delay in the rate of uptake of tracer via the kidney and in the time taken for the counts to reach a peak. The lesion may be confirmed by arteriography. Surgical correction has proved to be disappointing since blood pressure returns to normal in a small minority. An alternative non-

invasive technique consists of dilating the stenosis by means of a balloon catheter introduced into the renal artery under angiographic control. Investigations and operations should be reserved for those aged 35 years or less.

3 Conn's Syndrome

This results from an aldosterone-producing adrenal adenoma. The aldosterone results in reabsorption of sodium by the distal convoluted tubule in exchange for hydrogen ions and potassium. Patients present with mild to moderate hypertension without oedema. The diagnosis is suggested by a low plasma potassium and raised plasma bicarbonate. The hypokalaemia may result in muscle weakness and an inability of the kidney to concentrate; there is an increased liability to urinary tract infection. The diagnosis is confirmed by a raised plasma aldosterone in the presence of a low plasma renin activity. The hypertension responds to spironolactone, an aldosterone antagonist, but surgical excision of the adenoma provides a permanent cure.

4 Phaeochromocytoma

This results from a catecholamine-producing tumour of neuroectoderm, usually found in the adrenal medulla. It may occur in association with neurofibromatosis or multiple endocrine abnormality type II. The tumour may produce either adrenalin or noradrenaline, or a mixture, and the secretion may be continuous or paroxysmal. Hypertension may be sustained or paroxysmal in attacks when the patient becomes pale, sweats and may suffer from palpitations. The diagnosis is confirmed by finding an excess of hydroxymethoxy mandelic acid, a catecholamine metabolite, in the urine. The condition is treated by removing the adenoma surgically after the patient has been treated with first an alpha-blocker, such as phenoxybenzamine, and a beta-blocker such as Propranolol.

5 Coarctation of the aorta.

The mechanism by which this causes hypertension in the upper limbs is not completely understood. The diagnosis is suggested by the presence of a delayed femoral pulse when this is compared with the radial pulse. Collateral arteries may be readily palpable over the scapulae. A chest X-ray shows characteristic notching of the ribs by enlarged intercostal arteries. Surgical correction is only effective if the hypertension has not been sustained.

6 Cushing's disease

Hypertension occurs as part of this condition since the hormones produced have a mineralocorticoid action and result in sodium retention. Clinically, the patient has a Cushingoid habitus and the diagnosis is confirmed by raised plasma cortisol levels with loss of the diurnal variation. The blood pressure settles when the underlying condition is treated.

7 Renal parenchymal disease (see below).

The management of hypertension

The management should be along the following lines:

1 Exclude secondary causes (Table 14.1). An IVU is unnecessary unless there are proteinuria, erythrocytes (rbc's) in the urine, or renal impairment.

2 Assess the effect upon target organs (Table 14.2).

3 Treat the blood pressure. Good control of blood pressure reduces the excess mortality due to cerebrovascular accidents, renal failure and possibly myocardial infarction. Reduction in sodium intake and weight reduction if the patient is obese may be all that is required to reduce blood pressure. Where drug therapy is necessary a thiazide diuretic or a beta-blocker is usually the first choice. The two are used in combination where this is inadequate and, if necessary, a vasodilator such as hydralazine or prazosin is added. In exceptional cases one of the newer and more powerful agents may be necessary such as minoxidil (a powerful vasodilator) or captopril (an angiotensin-converting enzyme inhibitor).

MALIGNANT HYPERTENSION

Malignant hypertension occurs when there is extensive damage to the kidney, leading to arterial narrowing, which in turn leads to increased renin production. This exacerbates the hypertension and accelerates renal damage. The condition is rare and occurs in less than 1% of hypertensives; untreated it carries a 90% mortality at two years. Clinically the diastolic blood pressure is in excess of 130 mm of mercury. The fundi show haemorrhages, exudates and papilloedema, and urine testing reveals the presence of proteinuria. The characteristic pathological feature is the presence of arteriolar fibrinoid necrosis, especially in the kidneys. Biochemical examination confirms the presence of a raised blood urea and plasma creatinine.

Table 14.1 Causes of hypertension.

Cause	Mechanism	History	Examination	Biochemistry	Radiology	Other tests
Essential HT	Unknown	Non-specific family history	Non-specific	Non-specific	Non-specific	Non-specific
Renal artery stenosis	Renin secretion ↑ from hypoperfused kidney	Non-specific	Bruit audible over affected kidney	Non-specific	Affected kidney ⩽1.5 cm. in length than the contralateral kidney. Nephrogram delayed but more intense	Hippuran scan delay rate of uptake and rate of disappearance of tracer
Conn's Syndrome	Aldosterone secretion ↑ from adrenal adenoma	Weakness parasthesiae Polyuria	Non-specific	Hypokalaemic alkalosis Plasma aldosterone ↑. Plasma renin activity ↓	Non-specific or small tumour shown on angiography	Non-specific

					Chest X-ray	Confirmed by
Coarction	Uncertain	Non-specific	1 Femoral pulse delayed compared with radial pulse. 2 Collaterals palpable over scapulae	Non-specific	Chest X-ray shows rib notching	Confirmed by arteriography
Phaeochromo-cytoma	Catelacholamine producing adenoma of chromaffin tissue	Episodes of pallour, sweating, palpitations and hypertension	Non-specific ? Neurofibro-matosis	Raised urinary hydroxy-methoxy mandelic acid	Non-specific tumour may be seen on angiography	CT scan may show tumour
Cushing's Syndrome	Mineralocorticoid effect of hormones → sodium retention	Muscle weakness, thirst, polyuria	Cushingoid habitus	↑ Plasma cortisol	Non-specific	
Renal parenchymal disease	1 sodium and water retention 2 ↑ renin and angiotensin	Suggestive of renal disease	Stigmata of chronic renal failure	Blood urea ↑ and creatinine ↑	IVU shows damaged kidneys	

Table 14.2 Assessment of the effect of hypertension on target organs.

Target organ	Physical examination	Investigations
Retinae	↑ Light reflex A V nipping Haemorrhages and exudates Papilloedema	

Heart	Cardiac enlargement
	I V heart sound
	Heart failure
		C X R—cardiac
		  enlargement
		E C G—electrical criteria
		  of L V H S V_2 +
		  R V_5 ⩾ 35 mm

Kidneys	Proteinuria on stick
	  testing
		Raised blood urea and
		  creatinine

Malignant hypertension may be complicated by hypertensive encephalopathy in which there is drowsiness, transient neurological paresis, blindness and convulsions. Malignant hypertension is a medical emergency and the blood pressure must be brought down as soon as possible. However, overenthusiastic treatment resulting in hypotension may be dangerous since cerebral infarction and death may occur. Hydralazine in a dose of 20 mg or diazoxide in a dose of 75–100 mg, both by intravenous injection, are the drugs of choice.

Reduction of blood pressure in malignant hypertension often results in deterioration in renal function and occasionally anuria may occur. The G F R usually returns to pretreatment levels and in some patients even improves beyond them, but in some patients renal failure persists so that they require dialysis treatment.

Hypertension in renal parenchymal disease

In patients with renal parenchymal disease hypertension becomes increasingly more common and more severe as renal function deteriorates.

There are two principal mechanisms responsible:
1 increased renin production leading to an increase in angiotensin II;
2 sodium and water retention leading to an increase in blood volume.

In renovascular disease and in the early stages of renal glomerular diseases, ischaemia to the juxtaglomerular region leads to hyperreninaemia with the result that angiotensin II is produced in excess. Secondary hyperaldosteronism occurs leading to sodium retention. Normal homeostatic mechanisms are lost so that hypertension results, and this can be very difficult to treat. Beta-blocking agents and the angiotensin converting enzyme inhibitor captopril are appropriate drugs at this stage but as renal function deteriorates, other measures will have to be introduced.

Hypertension, whatever its cause, will, if untreated, accelerate the rate of deterioration in renal function and expose the patient to the real risk of cerebrovascular and myocardial catastrophes.

As indicated above, sodium retention plays a major role in the maintenance of hypertension in patients with renal failure. Sodium depletion is, therefore, an important part of treatment. Dietary sodium intake should be restricted to 50 mmol/day (no added salt) in mild to moderate hypertension and to 20 mmol/day in severe hypertension. In addition diuretics may be given to increase urinary sodium excretion. Thiazide diuretics will not produce significant natriuresis in patients with a GFR of less than 20 ml/min but loop diuretics (Frusemide and Bumetanide) work in those with GFRs as low as 3 ml/min. Large doses of diuretics may be necessary and patients should be warned of the potential hazard of dehydration; they should be instructed to guard against this by weighing themselves daily. If sodium depletion alone is inadequate, hypotensive agents such as beta-blockers, vasodilators (hydralazine, prazosin) or captopril may well be required.

Patients with interstitial nephropathies (chronic pyelonephritis, analgesic nephropathy, cystic diseases) are usually 'salt losers', i.e. they have high obligatory sodium excretion and are normotensive. Occasionally hypertension can accompany a 'salt losing nephritis' and this should be amenable to the wide range of hypotensive drugs available nowadays. If salt and water losses continue despite deteriorating renal function, extra sodium will be needed in the diet.

Chapter 15
Peritoneal Dialysis

This type of dialysis can be used for the treatment of renal failure or acute poisoning. It has the advantage of being simple to perform and requires no complicated apparatus, but the secret of its success lies in careful attention to detail.

Principle

Instead of an artificial membrane, the peritoneal membrane is used for dialysis. A physiological solution infused into the peritoneal cavity via a catheter will permeate through the whole of the space and will be in contact with 2–3 m² of potential dialysing membrane. The capillary blood traversing the membrane will exchange solutes with the dialysis fluid and many metabolic waste products like creatinine, urea, hydrogen ions and potassium will be removed when the fluid is drained off.

Unfortunately, the efficiency of the system is relatively low and so has to be continued for long periods of time, but as an emergency measure to remove excess extracellular fluid or to correct hyperkalaemia, it can be invaluable.

Technique

1 Empty patient's bladder.
2 Sterilize abdominal skin with iodine.
3 Select a site for the insertion of the catheter and anaesthetize locally. This site may be in the midline or in either flank.
4 Insert catheter and direct it towards the recto-vesical or recto-vaginal pouch.
5 Secure well to the abdominal wall and attach giving set.

Two litres of dialysate fluid in plastic bags are warmed to body temperature and infused into the peritoneal cavity, care being taken to eliminate air locks. It is conventional to add small quantities of heparin, e.g. 500 units, to the first few bags of fluid to prevent the formation of fibrin clots at the catheter tip.

After the infusion of dialysate fluid, it should be syphoned off immediately—the aim should be to complete each 2 l exchange in 1 hour.

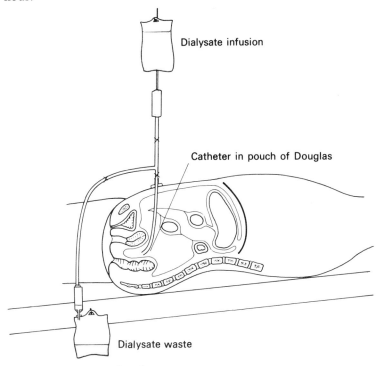

Fig. 15.1 Peritoneal dialysis.

Repeated exchanges should be continued until a satisfactory lowering of blood urea (less than 30 mmol/l) and creatinine (less than 500 μmol/l) have occurred and an appropriate amount of excess fluid has been removed. Thereafter, intermittent treatment can be continued.

Dialysis fluid

A variety of commercially prepared sterile solutions are available. Potassium is not included in these but has to be added prior to infusion according to the needs of the patient. Hypertonic solutions are available if excess fluid has to be removed (see Table 15.2).

Automatic dialysis machines

Much of the labour associated with changing dialysate fluid can be avoided by the use of an automatic recycling machine. A reservoir of fluid is pumped to a header tank, where it is warmed before infusion. Fluid balance is automatically monitored and the next cycle activated, according to the volume of fluid removed during the previous cycle.

Monitoring during dialysis

1 Measuring the input and output of peritoneal dialysis fluid is a useful guide to fluid balance, but the patient's weight should be checked at least twice a day. Actual weight loss is never as great as that indicated by the rough fluid balance chart.
2 Plasma electrolyte levels should be measured at least once per day, more often if there are problems with potassium and acid-base levels.
3 2-hourly blood pressure readings should be taken.
4 Daily culture of peritoneal effluent should be performed so as to detect infections at an early stage.

Table 15.1 Peritoneal dialysis.

Advantages	Disadvantages
Easy to set up and manage	Abdominal discomfort
Heparinization not necessary	Risk of abdominal injury
Disequilibrium unlikely	Immobility
	Pulmonary complications (e.g. pleural effusions and lower lobe collapse)
	Metabolic complication, e.g. hyperglycaemia, lactic acidosis and hypoproteinaemia
	Extravasation of fluid
	Expense

5 Plasma proteins should be measured every other day, for considerable protein loss can occur from the peritoneum. If hypoalbuminaemia becomes severe (<25 g/L) and hypotension develops, an intravenous infusion of protein should be given in order to maintain a normal plasma volume.

Management of complications

Prophylaxis

1 Active physiotherapy to minimize venous stasis and hypostatic lung problems.
2 A 60 g protein diet should be encouraged to offset transperitoneal protein and amino acid losses.

Special problems

1 Abdominal pain may be due to:
   (a) the use of hypertonic solutions;
   (b) peritonitis;
   (c) intestinal obstruction; or
   (d) perforation.
2 Retention of fluid due to:
   (a) malposition of catheter;
   (b) loculation of fluid by adhesions.
3 Metabolic
   (a) hyperglycaemia whilst using hypertonic fluid;
   (b) hypoglycaemia after stopping peritoneal dialysis;
   (c) lactic acidosis in patients with liver dysfunction;
   (d) hyponatraemia;
   (e) hypoproteinemia.

PERITONEAL DIALYSIS IN CHRONIC RENAL FAILURE

Although this was shown to be a useful form of treatment for patients with chronic renal failure, there were several practical problems to overcome. The two most important ones were those of the rigid catheter and infection.

Table 15.2   Peritoneal dialysis fluids—examples.

	mmol/l	mmol/l	mmol/l
Na*	130	140	140
Cl	90	101	101
Lactate	45	45	45
Glucose	1.36%	1.36%	3.86%
Ca*	1.8	1.8	1.8
Mg*	0.7	0.7	0.7

*Other concentrations of sodium, calcium, magnesium and potassium are available.

Tenckhoff overcame the catheter problem by producing a flexible model which could be fixed to the anterior abdominal wall by a dacron cuff.

The problem of infection has not been completely solved. Disconnecting and reconnecting containers of peritoneal dialysis fluid has always been a potential source of trouble. Boen (1961) was the first to use large sterile reservoirs of fluid with the aim of minimizing the number of connections and disconnections and subsequent developments in this field have been based on this system.

CAPD (Continuous Ambulatory Peritoneal Dialysis)

This has now become widely used as a definitive form of self treatment in chronic renal failure.

Instead of frequent exchanges of dialysis fluid, a bag of fluid is infused into the peritoneum and allowed to dwell there 6–8 hours, the connecting tube clamped and the patient going about his daily duties. At the end of the dwell period, the clamp is released, the empty bag lowered to ground level and the fluid drained off. The next 6-hour cycle is then started by the connection and infusion of a fresh bag of fluid. Bag exchanges can be performed by the patient at meal times and just before retiring at night, therefore there need be very little interference with daily living. Dietary restrictions are usually not necessary so that a good nutritional state is maintained and anaemia is usually only slight. Renal osteodystrophy may be less common than with other forms of treatment. Fluid retention is combatted by the intermittent infusion of a hypertonic solution.

Disadvantages

The revenue consequences of this treatment are quite high (£6000 per annum) but it is still cheaper than haemodialysis. The main problem is peritoneal infection, which must always be guarded against by good aseptic technique, and reporting of abdominal pain or the appearance of cloudy fluid. Prompt culture of the fluid and early treatment with antibiotics will prevent serious complications. As patients gain in technical experience, so the incidence of infection diminishes.

Advantages

Patients can be taught to perform dialysis in 2–3 weeks so that a long period of hospitalization is unnecessary. There is no expensive capital outlay and no modifications are necessary in the home.

It is a form of treatment that could well be very suitable for the elderly, the very young and the diabetic. As the peritoneum is very permeable to 'middle molecules' the general well being of the patient is likely to be better than with other types of dialysis.

Chapter 16
Haemodialysis

Principles

The principles of haemodialysis are very simple:

1 If blood is separated by a semi-permeable membrane from a physiological solution (known as the dialysis fluid), molecular particles will diffuse across the membrane passively from the compartment with the higher to that with the lower concentration. In the case of blood from a uraemic patient, urea, creatinine, uric acid, hydrogen ions, potassium and phosphate will diffuse into the dialysing fluid. Conversely, bicarbonate or acetate anions will pass from the dialysing fluid into the blood, thus correcting acid-base disequilibrium. The pore size of the membrane is designed so as not to allow large molecules such as proteins to pass through. It is this selective diffusion process that is termed **dialysis.**

2 If a hyperosmolar solution is used as the dialysis fluid, water will be removed from the blood by a process known as **osmosis.**

3 By applying a positive pressure to the blood compartment, or a negative pressure to the dialysis fluid compartment, water will pass through the membrane from the blood to the dialysis compartment. This is known as **ultrafiltration.**

By combining dialysis, osmosis and ultrafiltration, therefore, a fairly flexible form of artificial kidney can be designed. Consequently several forms of artificial kidneys have evolved over the past 30 years.

Coils

Tubular membranes wound around a rigid core, each turn of the coil being separated by a plastic mesh (Fig. 16.1).

Flat plates

Paired sheets of membrane separated by rigid or semi-rigid plastic plates (Fig. 16.2). In this way, blood passes between the membranes

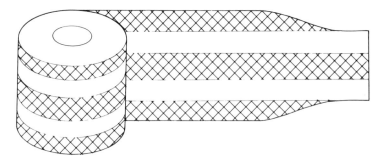

Fig. 16.1   Coil dialyser.

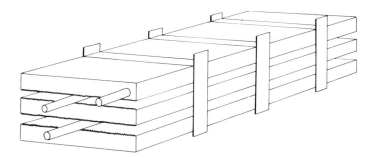

Fig. 16.2   Flat-plate dialyser.

whilst dialysis fluid flows on their outer surfaces. The original models were designed in such a way that they could be stripped and rebuilt after each dialysis. Nowadays a variety of disposable dialysers based on this principle are available.

Hollow fibres

Membranes can now be extruded in the form of fine hollow fibres, and a compact bunch of several thousand of these encased in a rigid tube (approximately 9 inches long) represents the latest models of artificial kidneys (Fig. 16.3).

The overall available dialysing area of an artificial kidney varies between 1 and 2.5 m², with an option for even smaller models for children. By technical developments, therefore, the compactness of

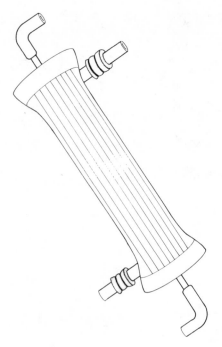

Fig. 16.3 Hollow-fibre dialyser.

design has reduced the size of artificial kidneys very considerably, so that portable dialysis systems are now almost a reality.

PREPARATION OF DIALYSIS FLUID (Dialysate)

This used to be achieved by mixing a large quantity of water with an appropriate mixture of salts.

Nowadays proportionating pumps will mix water and a solute concentrate continuously during the course of dialysis to make an ideal dialysis fluid without the need for large reservoirs.

A further advance in dialysis technology has been achieved by the use of sorbent cartridges introduced into the dialysis fluid circuit, so that a small volume of recirculating dialysis fluid can be purified immediately after being in contact with the dialysis membrane (Table 16.1).

Table 16.1 Example of composition of dialysis fluid.*

	Concentration (mmol l^{-1})
Sodium	130–135
Potassium	1.5–3.0
Calcium	1.6–1.8
Magnesium	0.25
Chloride	95–100
Lactate/acetate or bicarbonate	40
Glucose	0–10

*The exact composition can be varied according to the needs of the individual patient.

Access to the circulation

Prior to 1958, blood access for dialysis purposes was by repeated cannulation of peripheral arteries and veins, or via femoral vein catheters.

Shunts and fistulae

(a) In 1958 the Teflon shunt was devised. This was surgically implanted into a pair of peripheral vessels, e.g. radial artery and cephalic vein. When not in use, the shunt was bridged across by a silicone rubber connector (Fig. 16.4). It is usually called the Scribner shunt after its founder.

Problems of the teflon shunt

(a) Infection.
(b) Thrombosis.
(c) Accidental disruption.

(b) It was not until 10 years later that it was appreciated that surgically created arteriovenous fistulae in the limbs resulting in distension of the venous system were ideal for blood access. Once a fistula is established it can be repeatedly cannulated (Fig. 16.5) with little risk of thrombosis.

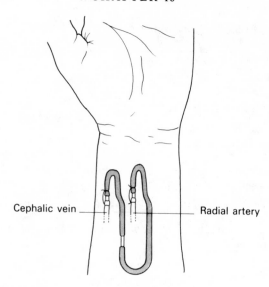

Fig. 16.4 Scribner shunt.

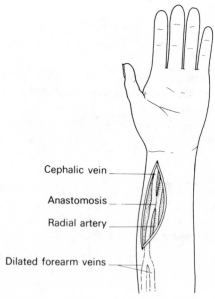

Fig. 16.5 Arteriovenous fistula.

Problems of arteriovenous fistulae

(a)   Infection.
(b)   Post-cannulation bleeding.
(c)   Progressive stenosis.
(d)   Aneurysm formation.

Subclavian cannulae

Recent interest has been aroused in the use of wide bore subclavian catheters introduced by the subclavicular route which can serve as vascular access for dialysis. Venous return can be achieved by another vein, or through the same or a double-channelled catheter. Scrupulous care should be taken to avoid infection.

Dialysis procedure

Dialysis treatment should be started before patients have developed crippling complications such as bone disease, pericarditis or peripheral neuropathy. This is not always possible because:
(a)   patients may have rapidly progressive disease and present for the first time in end-stage renal failure;
(b)   they may not always be referred to a specialized unit until moribund.
After the insertion of a subclavian catheter, a shunt or the establishment of an A V fistula, haemodialysis is the next step in the patient's treatment.

It is usual to start treatment by means of a series of short but frequent dialysis periods. In this way biochemical changes will be gradual and the patient is unlikely to suffer the consequences of too rapid alterations in the composition of his body fluids (the disequilibrium syndrome). After a week or so, the patient's treatment can be regulated to twice or thrice weekly treatment periods, each lasting for as long as is necessary (average 4-6 hours). As a general rule thrice weekly treatment keeps the patient in better health than twice weekly dialysis.

Home dialysis

Most patients can be trained to dialyse themselves at home. A training period of 6–8 weeks is usually sufficient to make them competent to needle their own fistulae, prepare the apparatus and monitor their progress on dialysis. Furthermore, they achieve greater independence, have a lower incidence of infection and their long-term survival is greater. The cost to the National Health Service is reduced by £5000, and space is made for another patient requiring dialysis treatment.

Patient selection

The majority of patients with chronic renal failure should be considered eligible for haemodialysis treatment. Certain technical and medical factors, however, mitigate against an overall satisfactory outcome in some cases.

1 Infants and small children. Technically, blood access is difficult, but more important is the fact that many of these children will not grow or mature resulting in many psychological problems.

2 Patients with severe cardiovascular or cerebrovascular disease may not benefit.

3 Severely diabetic patients with advanced retinopathy, peripheral vascular and cardiovascular disease generally do not respond well to dialysis.

4 Patients with hepatitis B antigen should be excluded from a dialysis unit because of the danger to other patients and staff.* They should be dialysed by trained staff in isolation and transferred to home dialysis as soon as possible.

5 Mentally subnormal and uncooperative patients.

Every new patient should be separately assessed from the point of view of responsibility and family support, and rather than have a rigid list of exclusive factors the doctor should be prepared to make certain allowances according to the circumstances.

---

*Hepatitis B immunization is now available for all high-risk staff and patients.

Diet

Once a patient is established on haemodialysis dietary restriction should be relaxed. A plentiful supply of protein should be encouraged (at least $0.75\,g\,kg^{-1}$ body weight/day) but there are a few important ingredients that should be carefully watched.

SODIUM

Hypertensive or fluid overladen patients must restrict salt intake until their blood pressure and cardiovascular status have returned to normal. Rarely, some patients may become salt depleted and will require sodium supplements.

POTASSIUM

The majority of patients with chronic renal failure have to limit potassium intake e.g. chocolate, toffees, dried fruit, coffee, wines, mushrooms etc. for in the absence of urinary output, they have no way of excreting potassium. Potassium is very toxic for it can cause serious cardiac problems if blood levels exceed $6\,mmol\,l^{-1}$.

PHOSPHATE

High plasma phosphate levels can lead to secondary hyperparathyroidism and serious metastatic calcification. Phosphate levels can be reduced either by restricting phosphate-containing foods, e.g. milk, cheese, eggs, or by taking aluminium hydroxide regularly (Unfortunately aluminium tends to make patients constipated so that laxatives may be necessary).

FATS

One of the commonest causes of death in the dialysis population is myocardial infarction. Hyperlipidaemia is common in renal failure and tends to be aggravated by a high carbohydrate diet. Sensible restruction of carbohydrates and saturated (animal) fats should be encouraged.

SUPPLEMENTS

Probably none is required provided dietary intake is adequate but most units give water soluble vitamins and folic acid. The need for iron is debatable.

Problems associated with regular haemodialysis

1　Blood access sites

Infection and thrombosis are the commonest problems. Ischaemia of fingers and toes may result from repeated unsuccessful attempts at cannulation. Attempts to dislodge clots from arterial and venous cannulae or fistulae may lead to pulmonary emboli. These are usually small and insignificant but occasionally an infected embolus may lead to a lung abscess.

Transient cerebral ischaemic episodes have been described as a result of vigorous irrigation of the arterial limb of a clotted Scribner shunt. These can be prevented by inflating a sphygmomanometer cuff to above arterial pressure proximal to the shunt.

2　Persistent anaemia

Modern dialysers have very small residual blood volumes after wash back, so that blood losses are minimal.

Chronic anaemia can usually be improved by intensive dialysis. Anabolic steroids, e.g. Sustanon, are sometimes valuable and blood transfusions should be reserved for those patients with symptoms such as angina of effort and heart failure.

3　Cramps

These occur not infrequently on dialysis and are probably due to sodium depletion. Increasing dialysis fluid sodium helps many patients; others benefit from oral sodium supplements during dialysis. If all measures fail, quinine sulphate (200 mg) usually gives relief.

4　Dementia

In centres where progressive stages of dementia have been observed amongst the dialysis population, high blood and tissue aluminium levels have been noted. The source of high aluminium levels is likely to be from the water (and therefore the dialysate supply). Aluminium is used intermittently, as an aggregating agent, in water supplies with high organic content; therefore the use of reverse osmosis to remove aluminium will protect the patients against this danger and, over a long time, will probably improve affected patients. The chelating agent desferrioxamine will bind aluminium and mobilise it from tissues, and reports of improvement in dementia have appeared. Successful renal transplantation similarly has a beneficial effect.

5 Hard water syndrome

In areas where the water is hard, softening or de-ionization is necessary before it enters the dialysis circuit—in this way, hypercalcaemia and hypermagnesaemia are avoided. Accidental breakdown in the water treatment plant can lead to acute hypercalcaemia resulting in tachycardia, hypertension, headaches, vomiting and abdominal pain. The plasma amylase level may be significantly elevated. If the fault is found and corrected, the patients rapidly improve when dialysed against a normal dialysate calcium concentration.

6 Peripheral neuropathy

Inefficient dialysis may result in a sensory neuropathy. This usually improves with intensification of dialysis.

7 Hepatitis

Outbreaks of hepatitis B infection are often associated with dialysis units. Infection usually occurs via the injection (accidentally or otherwise) of blood products, but as a result of their diminished immune responses the patients usually suffer only a mild transient illness. Hepatitis B surface antigens (HBs Ag) is normally cleared from the blood of patients within twelve weeks of their first symptoms, but in patients with chronic renal failure or on immunosuppression, the virus does not disappear and they become persistent carriers. They then remain a permanent hazard to the staff looking after them and to their families.

8   Osteodystrophy

Evidence for osteomalacia and/or hyperparathyroidism is usually present in patients with chronic renal failure (see Chapter 13).

9   Haemorrhagic pericarditis

This is a risk (usually when a patient first starts dialysis) for in severe renal failure a fibrinous 'uraemic' pericarditis can occur. If heparinization is not kept to a minimum during dialysis, quite severe haemorrhage may occur into the pericardium leading to tamponade. Nonsteroidal anti-inflammatory agents such as indomethacin are useful to alleviate the pain of pericarditis and helps to resolve the friction rub. When tamponade occurs, urgent paracentesis is called for.

10   Other haemorrhagic phenomena

Whilst patients are heparinized during the course of dialysis, spontaneous bruising is common, and if vigorous exercise is taken immediately after terminating dialysis, haemorrhagic joint effusions and muscle haematomata may occur.

11   Ruptured muscle tendons

Patients with osteodystrophy sometimes suffer tendon ruptures after only minimal stress—the quadriceps and Achilles tendons are the most commonly involved.

12   Impotence, amenorrhoea and loss of libido

These are common symptoms in dialysis patients and can lead to serious socio-psychological problems, including the breakdown of marital relationships. The problems are usually psychological and related to chronic ill health, loss of jobs, loss of confidence, etc. A sympathetic marital counsellor could have an important therapeutic part to play in these circumstances.

13   Psychological problems

Chronic ill health often leads to psychological stresses on family life. Dependence upon dialysis unit staff can lead to loss of initiative and shift of allegiance away from the family members. These problems can often be improved by transferring a hospital-based dialysis patient home. Even so, the restrictions of regular dialysis and diet prevent travel, particularly for holidays, and can lead to increasing resentment of the patient by the immediate family.

14 Cardiovascular complications

These account for more than 70% of deaths in patients on dialysis, with myocardial infarction particularly common. Cardiac failure or arrest from unknown causes (presumably hyperkalaemia) tend to occur in the younger age groups.

Prognosis

The overall European 10-year survival rate for haemodialysis patients is 50% with a wide variation between centres. The survival of patients on dialysis depends on many factors. Given a certain degree of competence on the part of the dialysing unit the patients' medical condition is the most important criterion. One can tentatively divide patients into good and bad prognostic groups.

Good prognosis

(a) Patients aged 10–55 years.
(b) Those without multisystem diseases.
(c) Normotensive patients or those with easily controlled hypertension.
(d) Emotionally stable and co-operative patients.

Poor prognosis

(a) Age over 65 years.
(b) Patients with multisystem diseases, e.g. diabetes, connective tissue diseases, amyloid, S.L.E.
(c) Patients with severe hypertension.
(d) Patients with severe atheromatous disease, e.g. cardiovascular, cerebrovascular or peripheral vascular.

(e) Emotionally unstable and unco-operative patients.
(f) Patients with malignant diseases, e.g. myeloma, carcinoma, etc.

The 5-year survival rate for the good prognosis group is of the order of 85% whereas that of the poor prognostic group is 30–40%.

Chapter 17
Renal Transplantation

Early attempts at renal transplantation in humans were between identical twins and close relatives, and the success rate was directly related to the closeness of this relationship. Non-related live and cadaveric donor kidneys failed badly, due to rejection and unsophisticated immunosuppressive therapy. The last 20 years, however, has seen great improvement in the results of both live and cadaveric kidney transplantation due to the following factors.

1 Improved pre-operative care which includes dialysis treatment and elimination of risk factors such as infection.

2 Available dialysis facilities to support patients with post-transplant oliguric renal failure.

3 Improvement in the quality of cadaveric kidneys and better preservation methods.

4 Improved use of immunosuppressive drugs.

Immunology

In all situations other than between identical twins, all cell membranes of grafted tissues, whether skin, bone marrow cells, kidney, liver, heart or lungs which are coated with antigens, are recognized as foreign by the host. They will therefore be destroyed by a process known as rejection.

This process of recognition is mediated by circulating small lymphocytes which relay the information to the reticuloendothelial system (R E S) (including the paracortical regions of lymph nodes) where transformation and division occurs, with the result that a generation of immunocompetent cells is produced. These can be differentiated into killer cells, immunoglobulin-producing (B) cells and memory cells.

The killer cells are thymus-dependent (T cells) and it is they that react with the target organ and initiate immunological damage.

B cells primarily produce immunoglobulins which react with foreign antigens and probably have other properties which aid T

171

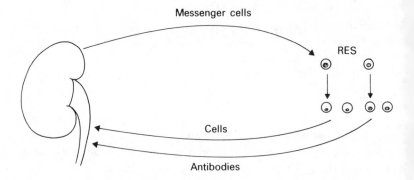

cell function. Patients who have been previously immunized against foreign antigens will react in an accelerated fashion when exposed to the same antigens subsequently—this is known as second set or hyperacute rejection.

ABO blood groups

ABO compatibility between donor and recipient is necessary, otherwise an accelerated form of rejection will occur. Rhesus blood group incompatibility probably does not matter.

HLA matching

Human leucocyte antigens (HLA) occur on the surface of most nucleated cells in the body and they can be detected readily in the laboratory on the surface of lymphocytes. Four HLA loci have been detected so far on the 6th chromosome—HLA-A, HLA-B, HLA-C and HLA-D. The HLA-A and B loci are normally the ones detected by a series of antisera derived from pre-immunized persons. Two antigens can usually be detected on each locus. Because of the time factor it is difficult to match for C and D antigens in cadaver transplantation. All transplant recipients are typed for HLA antigens prospectively so that the HLA profile of a prospective donor can be compared with a pool of recipients. The kidneys are then given to the best-matched recipients.

To exclude presensitized recipients, a direct lymphocytotoxic crossmatch should be performed between the recipient's serum and the donor's lymphocytes. As leucocytotoxic antibody titres fluctuate in any one person from time to time, regular testing is needed and serum samples with highest activity titres should be stored and used for direct crossmatching purposes.

Despite apparently well matched kidney transplants the outcome is not always predictable, and in many cases of apparent poor HLA-A and B matching, excellent results have been obtained.

The discovery of D locus antigens which are detectable on B cells only is likely to shed further important light on the subject.

In the case of live donor transplants between close relatives, HLA identity as well as a negative mixed lymphocyte reaction are desirable.

Selection of patients

Almost all patients accepted for regular dialysis treatment could be considered suitable for renal transplantation.

CONTRAINDICATIONS TO TRANSPLANTATION

1   Patients with systemic diseases such as oxalosis.
2   Patients with severe coronary artery or cerebrovascular disease.
3   Patients with active tuberculosis.
4   Patients with other active infection.
5   Patients with carcinoma.

Relative contraindications are:

1   Severely disordered lower urinary tracts, e.g. neuropathic bladders, fistulae, etc.
2   Severe diabetes mellitus, systemic sclerosis, etc.
3   HBs Ag positive patients.
4   Patients with active mesangiocapillary glomerulonephritis, focal glomerulosclerosis or active vasculitis because of the risk of recurrence in the transplant.

Selection of donors

Live donors

Only close relatives (usually siblings or parents) should be contemplated. If several fit siblings are available for consideration, the decision should be made according to HLA typing and mixed lymphocyte reactions.

Parental donors cannot be expected to be HLA identical with their offspring and the decision to use a parent's kidney will depend on other factors.

Cadaver donors

1 Should have no evidence of renal disease or any other disease that might affect the kidneys, e.g. diabetes, malignant hypertension.
2 Should be free from carcinoma (except intracranial tumours).
3 Should be under 65 years of age and previously healthy.
4 Should not be an H Bs Ag carrier.
5 Should not be infected.

Many potential donors die outside hospital so that little may be known of their previous state of health, therefore the decision as to whether or not the organs should be used may have to be made on very tenuous grounds. Testing a sample of bladder urine could prove a useful simple test under the circumstances.

Donors who die in hospital are usually easier to assess but if they are attached to life support machines they should be carefully monitored for infections, e.g. in upper respiratory tract, urinary tract and blood stream. If infection is present, adequate antibiotic therapy should be given prior to organ donation.

Removal of kidneys

This should be done by an experienced surgeon. As soon as the kidneys have been removed and found to be anatomically suitable for transplantation they are cooled by an intra-arterial infusion of a specially prepared solution at 4 °C. The time between the cessation of circulation and the commencement of cooling is known as the warm ischaemia time (WIT), and should be kept as short as possible.

Once cooled, they can then be stored for up to 24 hours if

necessary without significant further deterioration in cellular function. During this period—the cool ischaemia time (CIT)—they may have to be transferred to another hospital centre for transplantation.

It is always desirable to obtain permission from the next of kin of the deceased. When this is not possible the person in legal possession of the body may give permission. In the case of accidental death the coroner should always be consulted even if relatives have given permission. The law regarding procurement of organs after death varies in different countries.

Preparation of the recipient

Ideally, as renal failure progresses, careful dieting and the timely intervention of dialysis should pre-empt severe uraemic symptoms. Sources of infection are sought and they should be eradicated, if necessary, by the surgical removal of chronically infected organs, e.g. infected refluxing kidneys and ureters, bronchiectatic segment of lungs.

Barium meal or endoscopy and barium enema should be done to detect disorders such as peptic ulceration, oesophageal reflux, diverticular disease, etc., that might be aggravated by immuno-suppressive therapy. Appropriate therapeutic measures can then be taken prior to transplantation.

Micturating cystography may be necessary to determine the competence of the lower urinary tract of patients with a past history of outflow obstruction and/or vesicoureteric reflux. Abnormalities should be corrected prior to transplantation.

Fasting lipid levels should be measured and dietary advice given.

ABO grouping and HLA typing are done well in advance and it is generally felt that at least one blood transfusion should be given to the patient before transplantation.

Bilateral nephrectomy need not be performed routinely but reserved for patients with chronic urinary tract infections, analgesic nephropathy (because of the risk of malignancy), very large polycystic kidneys and rarely in patients with uncontrollable hypertension.

Post-transplant blood pressure control is usually better in patients who have previously undergone a nephrectomy operation.

TRANSPLANT OPERATION

The donor kidney is placed extraperitoneally in either iliac fossa (Fig. 17.1). At operation, the iliac vessels are first exposed and stripped of their adventitia. The donor renal artery is then anastomosed, either end-to-end to the internal iliac artery or end-to-side via a Carrel patch to the common iliac artery. The vein is joined end-to-side to

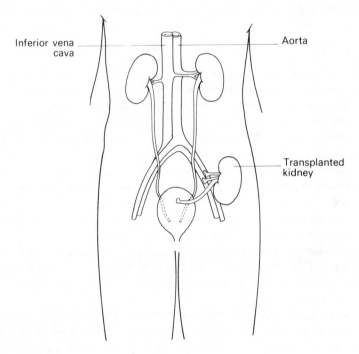

Inferior vena cava

Aorta

Transplanted kidney

Fig. 17.1 Position of transplanted kidney.

the external iliac vein. The ureter is then trimmed and implanted into the bladder wall through a submucosal tunnel or anastomosed directly to the lower end of the recipient's ureter.

As soon as the clamps are taken off the renal vessels, the kidney should perfuse uniformly with blood and acquire a healthy purple colour. It should be firm and within a few minutes a small amount of urine may be seen gushing from the ureteric orifice.

Immunosuppressive therapy

The early kidney transplant recipients were treated with radio-therapy, with or without corticosteroids. The usual result was bone marrow depression, intestinal destruction and infection leading to death.

6-mercaptopurine (6-MP) and, later, *azathioprine* were both found to be successful immunosuppressive agents in dogs and in man. Azathioprine has perhaps a wider therapeutic index than 6-MP and consequently it has continued to be used over the past 20 years. On its own, it is not very effective but given with corticosteroids, it has proved very successful.

Corticosteroids have anti-inflammatory properties, but they are also toxic to circulating lymphocytes and interfere with the synthesis of immunoglobulins. Their usefulness in immunosuppression is probably due, therefore, to a combination of these properties. Azathioprine is a purine analogue and consequently interferes with the synthesis of DNA in rapidly dividing cells. Unfortunately, the actions of steroids and azathioprine are not specific for the graft alone, so that bone marrow cells can be depressed and infections are common.

Antilymphocyte globulin promised to be a novel way of providing immunosuppression by inhibiting T lymphocytes, but unfortunately side-effects, such as thrombocytopenia and hypersensitivity reactions, limited its usefulness.

Many other agents have been tried experimentally and clinically, but without success. The latest agent used is cyclosporin A (a cyclic polypeptide antifungal agent) and initial results have been very encouraging. It has a specific action on lymphocytes and T helper cells are its main target. It also suppresses humoral immunity and prevents the release of lymphokines.

Immunological methods of inducing tolerance to the graft, and the use of enhancing or blocking antibodies are being investigated, but to date no consistently useful suppression of rejection has been produced.

Rejection

The interaction of donor organ and host is the most consistent phenomenon associated with transplantation. This is the so-called rejection phenomenon which varies in its intensity from patient to patient. It is not necessarily related to the degree of HLA matching as we understand it at present.

Evidence for rejection can be detected as early as a few days after grafting, and the tendency probably remains for the duration of the graft's existence. Most cases can be effectively suppressed by drugs, but with dire consequence in some patients.

Histopathologically, acute rejection can be classified as follows.

1   Minor mononuclear cell infiltration in perivascular distribution.
2   Confluent mononuclear cell infiltration sometimes infiltrating vessel walls.
3   2 plus interstitial haemorrhage, with or without evidence of renal tubular cell necrosis.
4   Deposition of fibrinoid material in arteriolar walls with thrombus formation in arterioles and glomeruli.

Chronic rejection, which occurs months or years after transplantation, is characterized by reduplication of the intimal layer of arteries, with consequent narrowing of the lumina, thrombosis, interstitial fibrosis and finally infarction of the whole organ. Glomerular capillaries also show thickening of the basement membrane and obliteration of the glomerular capillary lumina.

These grosser changes (3 and 4) along with chronic vascular occlusion are not usually reversible so that the kidney is best removed and the patient returned to the dialysis programme.

Hyperacute rejection

This rarely occurs if a negative cytotoxic crossmatch test is obtained prior to transplantation. However, if the kidney perfuses well after taking the vascular clamps off, and minutes later shows signs of intrarenal vasoconstriction with flaccidity and cyanosis, despite patency of the main renal artery, a biopsy is likely to show widespread haemorrhage due to vascular disruption and polymorphonuclear invasion of the glomeruli. There is no therapeutic advantage in leaving such an organ *in situ*.

Recognition of rejection

Clinically, rejection is relatively easy to detect if the kidney has functioned immediately after transplantation, for with any reduction in function not related to obstruction, septicaemia, urinary leakage or infarction, the most likely cause is rejection.

Where oliguric renal failure has developed as a result of ischaemic injury, the development of rejection can be quite insidious and clinical signs may be absent. Diagnosis can be difficult so that the following investigations may be helpful.

1 Isotope renography and gamma scanning.
2 Ultrasound of the kidney to exclude obstruction.
3 Renal biopsy.

Treatment

It is always necessary to give immunosuppressive drugs to the recipients of renal transplants (except in the case of identical twins). Up until 1978 the agents used were exclusively corticosteroids and azathioprine (Imuran). Antilymphocyte globulins and actinomycin C or D were also used in some departments.

The doses of steroids used varied widely, some authorities gave relatively large initial daily doses of prednisone or prednisolone (e.g. 60–100 mg day^{-1}) whereas others equally successfully used small doses (e.g. 20 mg day^{-1}). Where the larger doses were given at first, a gradual reduction to a maintenance dose of 10–20 mg day^{-1} was generally aimed at.

There is greater agreement over the dose of azathioprine which tends to be given in doses of 2–3 mg kg^{-1} day^{-1} depending upon the leucocyte and platelet counts. Where there is postoperative oliguria, the dose of azathioprine is kept at 1.0–1.5 mg kg^{-1} day^{-1}.

Since 1978 Cyclosporine A (CyA) has been introduced as an alternative to steroids and azathioprine with marked improvement in results. Approximately 30% of all transplants can be controlled by CyA alone, the rest usually require corticosteroid support. Initially CyA can be given intravenously in doses of 4 mg kg^{-1} day^{-1} with blood level monitoring and as soon as intestinal function has returned it can be given orally in doses of approximately 17 mg kg^{-1} day^{-1}. The actual dose should be determined according to blood levels and trough levels of 100–300 nm ml^{-1} should be aimed at, otherwise nephrotoxicity will develop.

All acute rejection episodes are treated by increasing the dose of steroids:
(a) either orally e.g. 200 mg prednisolone daily, then gradually reducing to the previous dose; or

(b) three daily intravenous doses of methyl prednisolone 0.5–1 g intravenously.

Early complications other than rejection during the first three months

Causes

1   Acute renal failure
  (a) Premortem hypotension or septicaemia in the donor.
  (b) Long warm ischaemic interval (>60 min).
  (c) Post-operative hypotension and/or septicaemia in the recipient.
  (d) Infarction of the kidney (arterial or venous).
  (e) Ureteric obstruction (oedema of ureter, stenosis, peri-ureteric haematoma, lymphocoele).
  (f) Ureteric leakage.
  (g) Nephrotoxicity from drugs, e.g. Frusemide plus cephaloridine, CyA.
  (h) Secondary haemorrhage from arterial rupture due to septicaemia.

2   Infections
  (a) Bacterial—wound sepsis, pneumonia and lung abscesses, urinary tract infections, meningitis, septicaemia.
  (b) Viral—*Herpes labialis*, ocular herpes, shingles, chicken pox cytomegalovirus hepatitis.
  (c) Fungal—candidal oesophagitis, aspergillus pneumonia and brain abscesses, cryptococcal skin and meningeal infections.
  (d) Protozoal—pneumocystis pneumonia.

3   Gastrointestinal
  (a) Acute peptic ulceration with haemorrhage or perforation.
  (b) Pancreatitis.
  (c) Diverticular abscesses and perforation.

4   Haematological
  (a) Leucopenia and thrombocytopenia.
  (b) Erythraemia.
  (c) Venous thrombosis and pulmonary emboli.

5   *Cardiovascular*
   (a)   Myocardial infarction.
   (b)   Cerebrovascular accidents.

6   *Diabetes Mellitus*
It can be appreciated that most of these early complications are related to the immunosuppressive treatment, so that very close observations of the patients and careful supervision of their drug therapy are important.

Late complications

Causes

1   *Bone and joint disease*
   (a)   Avascular necrosis in weight-bearing joints, such as the hips and knees, is relatively common. They are probably related to steroid therapy but the underlying mechanisms are not fully understood.
   (b)   Osteoporosis of the spine.
   (c)   Stress fractures—these may be a legacy of previous osteodystrophy.
   (d)   Autonomous hyperparathyroidism—a continuation of previous osteitis fibrosa.

2   *Infections*
The risk of infections remains whilst the patient takes immunosuppressive agents. Minor infections such as influenza and urinary tract infections are withstood without problems but bacterial and fungal pneumonias and tuberculosis remain a problem. Tuberculosis may be reactivated by immunosuppressive drugs but many cases of *de novo* infections have been reported. The incidence of long-term infections seems directly related to the total dose of steroids administered.

3   *Ocular complications*
Posterior central subcapsular cataracts not infrequently complicate patients on long-term steroid therapy. Glaucoma is also described.

4 Cardiovascular

Myocardial infarction is the second commonest cause of death in renal transplant patients. There is a high incidence of hypercholesterolaemia (type IIb hyperlipidaemia) in these patients and this has been thought to be related to the steroid therapy.

5 Malignancy

The incidence of lymphomas and cutaneous tumours is greatly increased in transplanted patients and may be due to altered immunological responses. Previously unsuspected tumours in the recipient have been observed to grow faster when immunosuppressed, and patients with cystic kidneys and analgesic nephropathy may be particularly at risk. Cutaneous malignancies occur most commonly in parts of the world where solar keratosis is common, e.g. Australia.

Tumours accidentally transplanted into recipients have been observed to proliferate whilst immunosuppressive drugs are given but to disappear if the treatment is discontinued.

6 Anaemia

A macrocytic anaemia may occur in long-surviving, immunosuppressed renal transplant recipients—this is thought to be related to azathioprine—it usually responds to a reduction in the dose.

7 Recurrent glomerulonephritis

It can be be very difficult to differentiate between the glomerular lesions resulting from chronic rejection and those due to recurrent glomerulonephritis. Clinically and histologically they may be indistinguishable. There is some evidence however that mesangiocapillary glomerulonephritis, focal glomerulosclerosis, Berger's mesangial IgA disease, H S P and rapidly progressive (crescentic) glomerulonephritis may be transmitted to the allograft.

Non-specific changes of 'transplant nephritis' can be seen in chronic rejection in patients where the original lesion was pyelonephritis or polycystic disease.

Clinically, the gradual deterioration in renal function with significant proteinuria and hypertension is typical of chronic glomerulonephritis or of transplant rejection, and gives an opportunity of taking a biopsy and comparing it light-microscopically, electron-microscopically and by immunofluorescence with a sample of the patient's own kidneys.

Results of transplantation

Between 1969 and 1981, over 33 000 renal transplants were performed in Europe and 43% of transplanted kidneys were still functioning at the date of survey. Comparison of 3582 grafts performed between 1974 and 1976 and 4487 between 1979 and 1981 showed 49% and 60% functioning grafts at 2 years. All patients were on steroids and azathioprine. Since the advent of Cyclosporin A, the 2 year functional survival rate has increased further to 76% and patient survival rate over a similar period was 88%.

Renal transplantation as a form of treatment of patients in terminal renal failure has much to commend it, for not only are the patients returned to the community to lead an independent life after the constraints of prior dialysis treatment, but they can now enjoy good health and return to gainful full-time employment.

Chapter 18
Renal Disease in Pregnancy

PREGNANCY AND THE NORMAL KIDNEY

During pregnancy, renal mass increases and calyces, pelves and urethra dilate. The cause of urinary dilatation is disputed.

Functional changes

Glomerular filtration rate and effective renal plasma flow are both increased by 30-50%. Increments are detectable within a few weeks of conception and are maximum during the second trimester. Levels return to normal after delivery. Blood urea, creatinine and uric acid levels are usually lower than in the non-pregnant woman, therefore, normal or high values of these substances will indicate substantial impairment in function.

Proteinuria. Normal pregnant women often have a little proteinuria and, if present beforehand, this is likely to be considerably increased during pregnancy, probably due to increased plasma flow. Compression of renal veins may contribute to the proteinuria late in pregnancy.

Body fluids. Total body water increases during pregnancy and plasma volume may increase by 50%.

Sodium. Gradual accumulation occurs during the course of pregnancy. As G F R is increased by 50% a massive increase in the amount of sodium filtered by the glomerulus and reabsorbed by the tubules occurs. Hormonal influences also play a part in determining the state of sodium balance.

Blood pressure. This, usually, is decreased and is minimal at 16-20 weeks. There is then a gradual increase up to term. Vasodilator substances such as prostaglandins are probably responsible. It is also known that plasma renin and angiotensin levels are high in pregnancy but the pregnant woman is resistant to their pressor effects.

Pregnancy has been described as a test of renal function. The main problems in pregnancy are due to the fact that X-ray investigations, such as intravenous urography and arteriography, are contraindicated and renal biopsies, though sometimes performed, are technically difficult and not without dangers. One is limited, therefore, to tests on the patient's blood and urine, with perhaps some assistance from ultrasonic and radioactive scanning departments.

In considering pregnancy in a patient with renal disease one must consider:

(a)   the possible effect the renal disease might have on mother and fetus;

(b)   the effect (if any) which the pregnancy might have on the mother's renal condition (Table 18.1).

Table 18.1   Effect of pregnancy on pre-existing renal disease.

Disease	Effect of pregnancy
Glomerulonephritis	No deterioration unless hypertension develops
Nephrotic syndrome ⎱ SLE ⎰	Well tolerated if under control
UTI	Infection more common, possible deterioration in function Watch BP
Polycystic kidneys	UTI frequent. Watch BP
Ureteric stones	Pass more easily
Ectopic kidneys ⎱ Pelvic kidneys ⎰	Well tolerated but may interfere with labour
Kidney transplant	Quite well tolerated. May need Caesarean section (CS)

Effect of renal disease on the mother and fetus

Special care of the pregnant mother with known renal disease goes without saying, but difficulties might arise where underlying renal abnormalities had not previously been suspected. This is why antenatal supervision is so important.

As a general rule, mild renal abnormalities as represented by proteinuria only, carry minimal risk to both mother and fetus, but the presence of hypertension and/or impaired glomerular filtration can cause a steep rise in fetal morbidity and mortality. The development of severe hypertension may also have an adverse effect on maternal renal disease. Advanced renal failure is usually associated with infertility, but occasionally conception occurs only to abort within the first twelve weeks. Rarely will a pregnancy survive to full term in such situations. It is usually claimed that toxaemia of pregnancy is common in patients with underlying renal disease, but it may be extremely difficult to distinguish between the two conditions. Clearly, any renal disorder brought to light during pregnancy should be followed up after parturition so that its nature can be clearly defined and further obstetric excursions planned well in advance.

GLOMERULAR DISEASE

Acute glomerulonephritis

Completely healed acute glomerulonephritis carries no added risk to pregnancy. However, if pregnancy occurs within two years of an acute glomerulonephritic episode, the risk of complications is said to be increased. Acute glomerulonephritis occurring *de novo* during pregnancy is very rare, and fetal mortality is very high.

Chronic glomerulonephritis

If proteinuria is the only index of glomerulonephritis no adverse effects on mother or fetus can be expected, but the association of hypertension carries a significant risk of fetal death. This is further increased if the glomerular filtration rate is reduced. There are reports of fetal mortality as high as 50% in cases where maternal blood urea levels were in excess of $8.3\,\mathrm{mmol\,l^{-1}}$.

Nephrotic syndrome

As in other forms of glomerulonephritis, the level of blood pressure and glomerular filtration rate are of paramount importance. The proteinuria and oedema can generally be managed with the help of diuretics and albumin infusions. Fetal dysmaturity often occurs when plasma albumin levels are low, so its maintenance at, or near, normal levels is very important.

The nephrotic syndrome, secondary to systemic diseases such as diabetes mellitus, S L E or P A N, have their own problems and fetal mortality is usually fairly high. However, if the underlying disease process is under control, e.g. with steroids, pregnancy is fairly well tolerated provided hypertension does not supervene.

Connective tissue disorders

Diseases such as S L E can, in some instances, be exacerbated during pregnancy but undoubtedly may show transient improvement. It is generally agreed, however, that in the puerperium severe relapses are common and if patients are taking steroids, an increase in the dose may be appropriate at this time. In polyarteritis nodosa and systemic sclerosis with renal involvement, the outcome of pregnancy is very poor in view of the likelihood of severe hypertension.

Urinary tract infections (see Chapter 10)

The incidence of asymptomatic bacteriuria in the pregnant population has been found to be 4–7%. The incidence appears to increase with age and multiparity. Several factors may be aetiologically important, e.g. ureteric dilatation and urinary stasis, renal glycosuria, potassium deficiency, endocrine factors and the presence of pre-existing renal disease.

The presence of bacteriuria in early pregnancy carries a significant risk of acute pyelonephritis (40%) and hypertension later in pregnancy, and adequate antibiotic treatment will prevent 75% of such attacks. Comparative studies have shown an incidence of acute pyelonephritis in 25% of untreated bacteriurics compared with 3% in treated patients.

The likelihood of prematurity in bacteriuric patients has been observed and this was shown to be more frequent in those whose infection was difficult to eradicate.

Patients with urinary infection are frequently hypertensive and so require careful treatment because of the increased danger of prematurity and fetal death.

Follow-up I V Us in bacteriuric patients after the completion of pregnancy have shown quite a high incidence of urogenital abnormalities. In patients whose urinary infections were difficult to eradicate urological abnormalities, not surprisingly, are more frequent.

Treatment

Pregnant patients should be screened for bacteriuria at their first antenatal clinic visit. Those showing significant growth of organisms (i.e. 10^5 ml^{-1}) should be given 7–10 days of antibiotic treatment to eradicate the infection. Initially a 'best guess' antibiotic such as trimethoprim or Augmentin should be started and changed if necessary when bacterial sensitivities are known. Thereafter, regular checks should be kept on urinary cultures throughout the duration of the pregnancy and further treatment given when indicated.

An alternative policy, and particularly appropriate in bacteriuric patients known to have scarred kidneys, would be to give a low-dose suppressive antibiotic regimen, e.g. nightly trimethoprim 200 mg after the completion of the initial course, and continuing for the duration of the pregnancy.

Urinary tract calculi

Stasis and infection in the urinary tract can predispose to stones. On the other hand, renal calculi may well be an important factor in patients with repeated infections, particularly with organisms of the *Proteus* species.

Dilatation of the ureters usually allows the asymptomatic passages of stones during pregnancy, but if they are arrested during their course down the ureter, the classical symptoms of colicky pain, nausea, vomiting, fever, dysuria and haematuria will occur. A single abdominal X-ray may be justified under the circumstances and a decision to operate or not will depend upon the size and position of the stone.

Acute renal failure

This is a well-recognized complication of pregnancy that is fortunately becoming a rarity, due to improved antenatal supervision and prompt correction of prerenal factors. Nevertheless, sepsis, haemorrhage and disseminated intravascular coagulation develop occasionally, resulting in oliguria which may need intensive dialysis treatment.

Though acute renal failure in pregnancy carries a relatively good maternal prognosis, severe damage to renal cortical tissue can sometimes follow an acute Schwartzman reaction associated with septic abortion or ante-partum or post-partum haemorrhage. Cortical necrosis is usually patchy and if the patient is dialysed, recovery with adequate renal function may eventually be achieved, though hypertension may remain a sequel.

Post-partum renal failure

This rare condition develops within six weeks of a normal pregnancy. The renal abnormalities are confined to the glomeruli and arterioles, and consist of diffuse necrosis, secondary to intravascular coagulation. The cause of this usually irreversible condition is not known and most patients require chronic haemodialysis.

Congenital renal diseases

Polycystic disease, ectopic kidneys and neurogenic disturbances are all potential sources of trouble during pregnancy, due either to infection or obstructed labour, therefore, careful monitoring of renal function and urinary cultures is vital.

Renal transplantation

Experience of pregnancy in this group of patients is growing annually. Though theoretically many problems might be envisaged, e.g. infection, hypertension, fetal adrenal insufficiency and fetal abnormalities, the majority of cases give no problems. Because of the pelvic position of the kidney, most cases are delivered by Caesarean section because of the risk of obstructed labour.

Toxaemia

No discussion of renal disease in pregnancy would be complete without some mention of this subject, because, for once, the kidneys are the victims and not the culprits of this condition. Although many factors probably play a part, the main renal features are related to the effects of disseminated intravascular coagulation, resulting in swelling of glomerular endothelial and mesangial cells and the deposition within capillary loops of fibrin—platelet microthrombi. These intrarenal changes may, in turn, contribute to salt and water retention and hypertension which are part of the syndrome of tox- aemia.

These glomerular lesions are usually considered to be completely reversible, but if severe enough, irreversible arteriolar necrosis may occur, resulting in persistent hypertension. Patients with underlying renal disease, including urinary tract infections, are reputed to be at increased risk from pregnancy toxaemia but, owing to the investi- gative constraints already mentioned, it is sometimes very difficult to distinguish between toxaemia and a worsening of the original disease.

Chapter 19
Surgical Aspects of Renal Disease

URINARY TRACT OBSTRUCTION

This may occur at any site between the kidney and the urethral meatus. As a result, the urinary tract above the obstruction becomes dilated and this is reflected up to the pelvis, calyces and tubules, the epithelium of which becomes flattened. If the obstruction is in or below the bladder then its wall becomes hypertrophied and trabeculated, and there may be bilateral ureteric dilatation.

Obstructive nephropathy

The term is given to the changes in kidney function which may occur with obstruction. There is a reduction in the nephron population which progresses with the duration of obstruction and this is manifest by a fall in the GFR. The higher the obstruction the more rapid is the rate of nephron death. In addition the tubules may not function normally so that the patient may be unable to form a concentrated urine. This is often not apparent during obstruction but when it is relieved there may be a dramatic diuresis which lasts for several days (see below). Finally a stagnant pool of urine above an obstruction is likely to become infected and once this has occurred it may be difficult to eradicate.

Clinically a patient with urinary tract obstruction may present in one of the following ways:

1 Acute renal failure can occur in a patient with only one functioning kidney which suddenly becomes obstructed.

2 Dull loin pain occurring because of dilatation of the ureter, pelvis and calyces. There may be exacerberbation when the patient drinks, for rapid dilatation of the pelvis occurs with the diuresis.

3 There may be episodes of severe loin pain known as Dietl's Crisis. It seems likely that the dilatation following a diuresis referred to in 2 results in the pelvis being further obstructed by an aberrant artery crossing the pelvi-ureteric (PU) junction. A dramatic rise in intra-

pelvic pressure results which can overcome the obstruction and relieve the symptoms.

4 Urinary tract infection which is difficult to eradicate.

5 Chronic renal failure is most commonly seen when the obstruction occurs in or below the bladder.

Causes of urinary tract obstruction

1 Pelvis

PELVI-URETERIC OBSTRUCTION

This occurs because of a muscular abnormality so that the peristaltic
waves in the pelvis are not transmitted into the ureter but rather the
junction becomes occluded by a sphincter type action. The patients
present with dull loin pain or attacks of Dietl's Crisis, but occasionally the pain may be referred more centrally so that the diagnosis is
difficult. Often urinary infection supervenes focusing attention on
the kidneys. The diagnosis will often be suspected from ultrasonic
examination, or an intravenous urogram where a dilated pelvis and
calyces with a normal ureter are seen. Confirmation is usually necessary and may be achieved by performing the I V U when the patient
is hydrated and taking films before and after an injection of Frusemide. The diuretic produces an increase in the size of the pelvis on the
affected side. Alternatively radionuclear scanning with and without
diuretics can give similar information. Rarely, antegrade pressure
flow measurements may be necessary pre-operatively. The results of
surgery are good if undertaken before irreversible nephron damage
has occurred.

Stones, blood clot, tumour and necrotic papillae may all cause
obstruction at the level of the pelvi-ureteric junction.

2 Ureter

INTRALUMINAL

1 Stones.
2 Tumour.
3 Blood clot.

4 Necrotic papillae occurring as a result of analgesic nephropathy, diabetes mellitus, sickle cell disease.

INTRAMURAL

1 Tumour, particularly transitional cell carcinoma (see below).
2 Stricture occurring as a result of tuberculosis, schistosomiasis or radiation therapy.

EXTRALUMINAL

1 Tumour.
2 Aberrant blood vessels.
3 Pregnancy.
4 Retroperitoneal fibrosis. This may be idiopathic (considered by some to be a form of perivasculitis) and associated with mediastinal, thyroid and penile fibrosis. This condition is associated with a high ESR. Drugs such as methysergide (antiepileptic) are known to be aetiological agents. Malignant tumours of the retroperitoneal tissues or infiltrative tumours arising from the prostrate or bladder can cause a similar clinical picture.

The diagnosis is suggested by IVU showing dilation of the upper tracts with medial deviation of the ureters. Retrograde catheters pass up the ureters without difficulty but contrast does not descend because of lack of ureteric peristalsis.

Treatment depends upon aetiology, so a biopsy is always desirable. In benign retroperitoneal fibrosis, ureterolysis with or without steroids is recommended. In the case of malignant infiltration from prostatic carcinoma hormonal treatment, Honvan, for example, may be appropriate.

3 Bladder and urethra

(a) Carcinoma of the bladder (see p. 199).
(b) Enlargement of the prostrate (benign or malignant). The patient may present in the following ways.

   1 Delay in initiating micturition, poor stream and terminal dribbling.
   2 Acute retention occurring after a period of high fluid intake.
   3 Retention with overflow and dribbling incontinence. Often,

probing with the finger alone will distinguish between a benign and malignant prostatic enlargement since the latter is hard, irregular and there is loss of the median sulcus. Confirmation may be obtained by needle biopsy and there is probably no indication for performing an acid phosphatase. There is no need to perform an intravenous urogram in every patient with prostatic enlargement since it is unlikely to provide useful information regarding renal function or morphology. If the GFR is reduced a period of catheter drainage in order to allow for recovery of renal function and correction of electrolyte disturbances should be recommended. Carcinoma of the prostate is a common condition and is often an incidental finding at post mortem or at histological examination of prostatectomy specimens. Of all the patients with this condition only a minority will die from the results of the malignancy so that treatment is reserved for those patients with symptomatic metastases which can be controlled by orchidectomy, hormone therapy (Stilboestrol 1 mg t.d.s.) or by local radiotherapy.

(c) Vesical calculi. These tend to develop *in situ* and occur in patients who have difficulty in emptying their bladder; if renal calculi are able to negotiate the ureters then under normal conditions they will manage the rest of their journey to freedom without difficulty. Patients present with frequency of micturition, dysuria and suprapubic discomfort which is relieved when they lie flat. Infection may supervene. The calculi are usually radio-opaque so that they may be seen on a plain X-ray. Small stones are treated by crushing them with a special instrument (lithotome) so that the fragments may then be washed out. Large stones have to be removed through a formal cystotomy.

(d) Neurogenic bladder. This may occur because the bladder becomes denervated, or the pathway between the bladder and the spinal cord is interrupted. In this situation the bladder becomes distended and emptying may only be achieved by resecting the bladder neck. The patient is then able to void by increasing intra-abdominal pressure but the operation may lead to incontinence. Where the higher pathways in the spinal cord are affected following trauma, spinal tumour, multiple sclerosis, etc., the bladder wall undergoes continuous contractions leading to hypertrophy of the walls. Often this takes place against a closed sphincter so that a bladder neck resection may also be advisable. Where such an operation fails to control the situation an indwelling catheter may be necessary. In these circumstances infection is inevitable and antibiotic therapy should be reserved for systemic illness only. Haematuria or heavily infected urine containing debris may be controlled by bladder wash-outs with saline or chlorhexidine.

Intermittent self-catheterization has been shown recently to be a more acceptable form of treatment than continuous catheterization.

TUMOURS OF THE KIDNEY

Adenocarcinoma of the kidney (Grawitz tumour or hypernephroma)

More common in males than females. Incidence increases with age.

Morphology

The tumour usually arises in the upper pole of the kidney. Bilateral tumours occur in 5% of patients. Macroscopically, the tumour is a spherical mass of bright yellow/grey tissue which distorts the renal outline. There is often a distinct pseudo-capsule and the tumour tissue may break down, giving rise to cyst formation. Micro-scopically, they are very pleomorphic with some cells resembling tubular epithelial cells, others appearing solid—the so-called clear cells. Metastases occur mainly by the blood stream to the lungs, but local lymphatic spread to liver and bone and local invasion can also occur.

Clinical features

These are slowly growing tumours and may present late. The three commonest forms of presentation are:
1 haematuria either micro- or macroscopic;
2 pain in the flank;
3 a palpable mass in the flank.

In addition renal adenocarcinomata may give rise to numerous other phenomena as follows:
(a) pyrexia (a renal tumour should be considered in a differential diagnosis of anyone with a pyrexia of unknown origin (PUO));
(b) hepatosplenomegaly with a non-specific hepatitis;

(c)   normochromic, normocytic anaemia and raised ESR;
(d)   endocrine abnormalities
  (a)   polycythemia secondary to raised erythropoietin production
  (b)   hypertension
  (c)   hypercalcaemia due to either bony secondaries or excess production of a PTH like substance
  (d)   Cushing's syndrome due to ectopic adrenocorticotrophic hormone (ACTH) production;
4   neurological abnormalities including peripheral neuropathy;
5   secondary amyloidosis;
6   glomerulonephritis due to anti-tumour antibodies;
7   heart failure due to the vascularity of the tumours;
8   vena caval obstruction;
9   the diagnosis should be considered in a patient who acutely develops a varicocoele on the left side. This occurs where there is venous spread of the tumour into the left renal vein into which the testicular vein drains.

Investigations

Where a renal adenocarcinoma is suspected an IVU should be performed, since it is likely to be diagnostic in 95% of the cases. The following signs may be found.
1   Calyceal distortion with displacement, elongation or compression. In these circumstances the differential diagnosis rests between a malignancy or a simple cyst. Usually these may be distinguished by an ultrasound examination but where doubt exists aspiration of the cyst with cytological examination may be necessary.
2   There may be loss of renal outline on tomography where the tumour has spread outside the renal capsule.
3   The renal tissue may be non-functioning so that no nephrogram develops. This may occur because of either arterial or venous occlusion, obstruction to the pelvis or ureter or massive destruction of the nephron mass.

If a tumour is strongly suspected after IVU an arteriogram should be undertaken.
(a)   To exclude a tumour on the other side (5% of cases).
(b)   To delineate the anatomy of the arteries on the affected side.
(c)   To visualize the renal vein or inferior vena cava during the

venous phase of the examination to see whether the tumour has spread into them. Where a good venous phase is not obtained on arteriography a venogram may be helpful. Additional information may be obtained by ultrasound examination. If available, CT scanning will usually give sufficient information without having to resort to arteriography.

Treatment

For unilateral tumour, nephrectomy is the treatment of choice even if metastases are present, for the latter may regress subsequently. Solitary metastases, e.g. in lung or brain, may be worth removing as they could represent a single embolic episode. The prognosis for this tumour does not seem to be influenced by tumour spread outside the renal capsule or into the renal vein. Local lymphatic spread, however, carries a very poor prognosis. In the case of bilateral tumours, resection of the lesions may be possible with conservation of normal renal tissue. This may require bench surgery and re-implantation into an iliac fossa. If the tumours are not resectable, bilateral nephrectomy and long term dialysis would be appropriate.

Unfortunately, hypernephromata do not usually respond to chemotherapy or irradiation, but it is claimed that up to 20% of patients with painful metastases may improve symptomatically with hormone treatment such as medroxy progesterone acetate (Provera).

Prognosis

If the tumour is confined to the kidney the 5-year survival rate is 60%. Overall survival rate is 36–50% at 5 years and 17–28% at 10 years.

Nephroblastoma (Wilm's Tumour)

Incidence

This is a tumour which has a peak incidence at 18 months of age, and in 75% of cases occurs before the age of 3 years. Like the adenocarcinoma of adults it is bilateral in 5% of cases. It is twice as common in boys as in girls. Since it may occur in children who have congenital abnormalities such as hemihypertrophy or urogenital malformations it seems likely that it is the result of some agent which is both oncogenic and teratogenic. It spreads locally to adjacent tissues and metastasizes to the lungs, liver, bone and brain.

Morphology

The tumour is homogeneous and pale but the centre may become necrotic, haemorrhagic and cystic. The pseudo capsule is much less apparent than with the adenocarcinoma. Microscopically, the picture is extremely variable with predominant primitive spindle cells and round cells, but some form of mesodermal tissue may usually be recognized.

Clinical features

The most constant presenting features are a palpable abdominal mass, hypertension, pain and haematuria. Ascites and oedema may result from I V C compression. Often the child appears ill and wasted. Also like the adenocarcinoma endocrine abnormalities, pyrexia, anaemia, etc. may all occur.

Differential diagnosis

Hydronephrosis, unilateral cystic disease of the kidney and neuroblastoma are the main differentials.

Investigations

The investigations follow the same line as in the adult except that an arteriogram may be more difficult and potentially more dangerous in young children. CT scanning should obviate these unpleasant investigations.

Treatment

Nephrectomy is performed but, unlike the adenocarcinoma, the adrenal and surrounding fascia should be removed. It is arguable whether the aortic nodes should also be excised. Radiotherapy and chemotherapy in the form of actinomycin D or vincristine improve the prognosis, but it is uncertain whether this should be given as pretreatment or adjuvant therapy. In those treated before the age of one the prognosis is excellent, but it is still extremely good in those over this age. Where the interval of follow up exceeds the child's age at the time of operation then Collin's law is satisfied and the child may be considered cured.

Tumours of the renal calyces, pelvis, ureters and bladder

These tumours may appear anywhere in the urothelium, may be multiple in up to 60% of cases and may even appear bilaterally. The tumours may be papillomatous, solid or give rise to ulceration. Histologically they may be either transitional cell tumours or squamous cell carcinomas.

Aetiology

These are more common in males than females and occur mainly in the 60–70 year olds, but are seen in most age groups. The tumours were found to be common in those working in the chemical industry, dyeing and rubber trade where it has been shown that naphthylamine and benzidine are the carcinogens. Tumours are more common in those who smoke and are also seen in those with bilharzial infection (*Schistosoma haematobium*) where the tumour is also a squamous cell carcinoma. Patients who have analgesic nephropathy have a much higher incidence of urothelial tumours and there is an increased instance in those with leucoplakia or bladder stones.

Clinical features

Tumours of the urothelium give rise to haematuria which may be macroscopic and severe enough to lead to anaemia. Where there is occlusion to the ureter hydronephrosis may develop, giving rise to loin pain. Urinary tract infection may supervene and dysuria is common.

Investigations

Any patient presenting with haematuria should have an intravenous urogram and a midstream specimen of urine sent to the laboratory to confirm the presence of red cells and to exclude infection. It is now possible to differentiate glomerular bleeding from that arising more distally by means of phase contrast microscopy. Patients who are shown to have haematuria of non-glomerular origin even in the presence of a normal IVU should be referred to a urologist for cystoscopy. Where a urothelial tumour is suspected it is possible to examine the urine cytologically. For the examination a *fresh specimen* is required, preferably after the patient has drunk about a litre of water and taken vigorous exercise so that the cells are agitated into the bladder. Unfortunately, this investigation may give false positives in those with stones or inflammation, and false negatives where the tumour is well differentiated. At cystoscopy it may be possible to biopsy the tumour if it is in the bladder, or to obtain material for cytological examination by ureteric brushings.

Treatment

Where the tumour is in the calyx, pelvis or ureter then a nephroureterectomy should be performed and a cuff of bladder removed. Bladder tumours should be considered potentially invasive carcinomas, however apparently benign their histology. Surgical resection is undertaken to obtain adequate material for histology and to stage the tumour. Further resection is necessary where there is evidence of recurrence. Radiotherapy is reserved for those with invasive tumours.

Adenomata

These are the commonest benign tumours of the kidney. They are small and are composed of small uniform epithelial cells. Pre-operatively they are indistinguishable from hypernephromata. They cause no symptoms and are found usually at post mortem.

Adenomyolipomata (hamartoma)

These occur in association with tuberose sclerosis. They are composed of smooth muscle, fat and angiomatous tissue. They can be difficult to differentiate from renal cell carcinomas.

Haemangiopericytoma (juxtaglomerular tumour)

These are very rare and are the site of excessive renin production with resulting severe hypertension. If found and removed, the hypertension is likely to be cured.

Fibroma, leiomyoma and neurogenic tumours

Fibroma, leiomyoma and neurogenic tumours are very rare but may reach considerable size.

Metastatic tumours

Lung and breast cancers usually metastasize to the kidneys. Rarely do these metastases give rise to any renal symptoms or functional abnormalities.

Chapter 20
Drugs and the Kidney

When drugs are administered to patients they are absorbed into the blood stream and are transported to various parts of the body where they exert their pharmacological effects. During their period within the body they are themselves subjected to complex metabolic and excretory events.

The pharmacological effect of a drug on the patient depends upon several factors.

1   Route of administration

Drugs given by mouth are swallowed and absorbed from the gastro-intestinal tract into the portal system where they are transported to the liver and further processed. Drugs administered parenterally or sublingually will enter the venous systemic circulation and are capable, therefore, of exerting their pharmacological effect without first having to pass through the hepatic circulation.

2   Protein binding

The pharmacological availability of any drug will depend on how closely it is bound to protein and other tissues. The degree of binding will depend on the concentration of the drug, the number of available binding sites and the affinity of that particular drug for those sites. Normally, a dynamic equilibrium occurs between bound and un-bound drugs so that a reduction in free chemicals will lead to a shift in the dissociation from the bound state. In renal failure, protein binding may be diminished because of fewer binding sites. Drugs may also compete with each other for these sites.

3   Degree of liver metabolism

Orally administered drugs pass through the portal system into the liver where they are processed by microsomal enzymes of the smooth endoplasmic reticulum. Chemical structure of drugs is sometimes altered by acetylation or oxidation and they may be bound to substances, thus increasing solubility and excretion via the biliary system. Liver enzymes may be inhibited by a degree of renal impairment.

4   Distribution of drugs throughout the body

This depends upon the physicochemical properties of the drugs, their water or fat solubility and their degree of ionization. Fat soluble drugs will usually pass through cell membranes rather easier than water soluble drugs.

5   Elimination of drugs

This is primarily a function of the kidneys and is achieved either by glomerular filtration or tubular excretion.

The glomerular filtration of any substance will depend upon the glomerular filtration rate, the blood level of the drug, its solubility and the degree of protein binding. Tubular excretion is more complex. Ionized substances entering the luminal fluid will tend to remain in solution and be excreted in the urine. The rate of excretion can be enhanced by adjusting the pH of the urine, e.g. weak bases can be excreted more quickly by rendering the urine acid, whereas weak acids would be excreted more rapidly by adjusting the pH to the alkaline side. Drugs that are less well ionized tend to diffuse back into the tubular cells and this is enhanced if their lipid solubility is high. Tubules, in addition, have active secretory mechanisms, one for organic acids, the other for organic bases. These are both active transport systems.

Effects of drugs on the kidney

Not only do the kidneys play a vital part in the excretion of drugs, but one has to remember that they may be important target organs for the action of drugs as well. This may be intended (for instance in the use of diuretic agents) but on the other hand it may be an undesirable consequence brought about by potentially toxic drugs or in the face of declining function, by the excessively high blood levels of drugs and their metabolites. Special care must always be taken, therefore, when such drugs are prescribed. Kidneys also have a role to play in the metabolism of vitamin D, and failure of kidney function leads to a defective synthesis of active vitamin D metabolites.

Kidneys are susceptible to the toxic effects of drugs and chemicals because of the following reasons:

1 They have a rich blood supply.

2 The renal medulla is hypertonic and the site where drugs are concentrated.

3 When renal function is impaired, drug levels in the blood will accumulate.

4 In the presence of renal failure, hypersensitivity reactions with consequent vasculitis are not uncommon.

5 The rate of metabolism of drugs is often slower in the face of declining renal function.

DRUG TOXICITY

The consequences of drug toxicity on the kidneys often simulates spontaneously occurring renal diseases, e.g. renal failure, nephrotic syndrome, S L E-like syndromes, renal tubular disorders, electrolyte and metabolic disturbances, neoplasia and stone formation.

Acute nephrotoxicity leading to renal failure

The vascular system, the nephron and the interstitial tissues are potentially vulnerable to the action of toxic agents. Some drugs are capable of attacking more than one part of the system simultaneously.

1   Antimicrobials

These are probably the widest group of drugs used in clinical practice these days. Some knowledge of their metabolism and excretion is desirable if one is to avoid the problems of toxicity.

SULPHONAMIDES

These are normally acetylated by the liver and excreted by the kidneys. Some are relatively insoluble substances and can cause tubular and ureteric blockage unless a high fluid intake and alkalinization of the urine is practiced. Hypersensitivity vasculitis has also been ascribed to these drugs.

PENICILLINS

Most preparations are relatively non-toxic but methicillin occasionally produces hypersensitivity glomerulonephritis, with proteinuria and an S L E-like syndrome.

CEPHALOSPORINS

Cephaloridine, particularly when used with frusemide, can produce renal tubular damage. The newer generations of cephalosporins are less toxic.

TETRACYCLINES

These anti-anabolic drugs can raise the blood urea in patients with diminished renal function. Outdated tetracycline preparations have been reported as producing a Fanconi-like syndrome with hypokalaemia. Vibramycin (doxycycline) is the only safe tetracycline to use in renal failure because of its high protein binding.

AMINOGLYCOSIDES

These are all potentially nephrotoxic and ototoxic. Great care is needed in their use in patients with renal failure and blood levels should be measured.

POLYMYXINS AND COLOMYCIN

These are both nephrotoxic and neurotoxic.

VANCOMYCIN

This is also nephrotoxic and can produce proteinuria.

RIFAMPICIN

This can cause hypersensitivity interstitial nephritis with tubular necrosis.

AMPHOTERICIN B

This is an antifungal agent which produces proximal and distal tubular damage with consequent hypokalaemia.

2   Anticoagulants

Phenindione has been described as producing hypersensitivity glomerulonephritis.

3   Anaesthetic agents

Methoxyflurane is metabolized in the liver and releases fluoride radicles which can cause distal tubular damage. Calcium oxalate crystals tend to be deposited in the renal tubules.

4   Radiographic contrast media

Intravenous contrast media such as Telepaque and Biligrafin, used in cholecystography, may cause renal damage, particularly in patients who have compromised liver function and are jaundiced. These drugs seem to be more dangerous if given within 24 hours of an oral cholecystogram and this danger seems to be enhanced by dehydration.

Renal contrast media have also been implicated as causing renal damage in patients with diabetes mellitus, myeloma and amyloid disease but provided the patient is kept well hydrated, the danger seems to be minimal.

Table 20.1   Drugs toxic to the kidneys.

Toxicity	Drug
Vasculitis	Sulphonamides, methicillin, thiazides, allopurinol
Glomerulitis	Hydralazine, penicillamine, sulphas, phenindione, troxidone, heavy metals
Tubular and interstitial damage	Aspirin/phenacetin, sulphas, methoxyflurane, allopurinol, biligrafin, rifampicin, septrin, phenylbutazone, dextrans
RPF	Methysergide, ergotamine

Systemic lupus-like syndrome

Patients who are phenotypically slow acetylators are susceptible to this type of complication if exposed to hydralazine, isoniazid, procainamide, phenytoin, methyldopa, phenylbutazone and penicillamine. The clinical pattern of SLE with positive antinuclear factor (ANF) can occur. Renal involvement develops in some cases. Improvement may occur if the drugs are discontinued.

The nephrotic syndrome

Membranous glomerulonephritis has been recorded following treatment with certain drugs, e.g. tolbutamide, penicillamine, captopril, probenecid and troxidone. Gold salts given to patients with rheumatoid arthritis may also produce heavy proteinuria but an awareness of this complication should stimulate regular urinalysis and the withdrawal of the drug at the first sign of proteinuria. The mechanism of drug-induced nephrotic syndrome is probably antigen-antibody mediated, the drug acting as a hapten and attached to a carrier protein.

Retroperitoneal fibrosis (RPF)

This has been described in patients taking methysergide, ergotamine, hydralazine and methyldopa and can lead to ureteric obstruction. The aorta, inferior vena cava (IVC), mediastinal structures, liver and thyroid may also be involved.

Analgesic nephropathy

Chronic ingestion of compound analgesic tablets can lead to an interstitial nephritis and papillary necrosis. The condition is commoner in certain countries than others, e.g. Australia and Switzerland. Women are affected more often than men; they usually take analgesics to alleviate intractable pain and are often anaemic and dyspeptic. The renal damage is probably due to medullary ischaemia and tubular damage with obstruction. Superimposed infection is not uncommon. Necrotic papillae calcify and may slough off, resulting in ureteric obstruction. If the analgesic drugs are stopped, it is claimed that the condition does not progress. Moreover, transitional cell tumours have been reported as a complication of this condition.

Interstitial nephropathy

Drugs which cause potassium depletion such as diuretics, amphotericin B and laxatives can produce interstitial and tubular damage resulting in fibrosis. Hypercalcaemia from vitamin D intoxication can result in similar changes with the added problem of calcification.

Uric acid nephropathy

This may occur spontaneously in gout, and is well recognized in patients treated for neoplastic disease such as lymphoma and leukaemia. Due to the breakdown of nucleic acids, a massive uric acid load is put on the kidney which can sometimes lead to tubular and ureteric obstruction. An awareness of this complication can be pre-empted by the use of allopurinol and ensuring a high alkaline urine output.

Prescribing for patients with renal diseases

The following questions need to be borne in mind:
1 How is this drug excreted?
2 What are the likely toxic effects of the drug?
3 How well bound is the drug to protein?
4 Does this drug produce abnormal sensitivity reaction in patients with renal failure?
5 In the case of urinary infections, will the drug be excreted in sufficient concentration to be effective?

Points to remember

1 Renal function must be assessed before planning drug regimens.
2 Nephrotoxic drugs should be avoided in the presence of renal disease.
3 If you have to use a potentially nephrotoxic drug, make sure that blood levels are measured regularly. If the patient is on dialysis, it would be very important to know whether the drug is dialysed or not. As a rule, water-soluble drugs that are well excreted by glomerular filtration will be dialysed out. Dose adjustment will, therefore, have to be made depending on blood levels in renal failure, and as renal function diminishes. This can be achieved by either using

reduced amounts of drug at conventional time intervals or giving the same dose at longer intervals. Either method is acceptable, though better therapeutic levels can be achieved by the latter method. If a drug is known not to be excreted by the kidneys, then it is usually safe to be used in normal doses, e.g. erythromycin and fucidic acid. In the case of urinary tract infections, it is important to establish that the drug is well excreted in the urine, even in the face of diminishing renal function. Trimethoprim, cephalexin and penicillin derivatives are usually adequately excreted in the urine even in renal impairment, and their dosage should probably not be reduced. Nitrofurantoin and nalidixic acid should never be used as they are poorly excreted and are potentially very toxic.

Diuretics, apart from frusemide and bumetanide, are fairly ineffective at glomerular filtration rates of less than 20 ml min^{-1} and there is little to be gained by persisting with them. Potassium-conserving diuretics such as spironolactone, triamterene and amiloride should not be given to patients with poor renal function.

Hypotensive agents

Beta-blockers, hydralazine and prazosin are usually safe and modification of the dosages is not usually necessary. Other agents, such as minoxidil and captopril, also seem to be suitable in renal failure but dose adjustment may be necessary.

Antidiabetic drugs

Insulin requirements usually diminish as renal failure advances. Oral hypoglycaemic drugs should be avoided if possible. The biguanides, phenformin and metformin can cause severe lactic acidosis.

Organic solvents and herbicides

Carbon tetrachloride, ethylene glycol and paraquat are all potentially nephrotoxic and usually produce severe tubular necrosis. Carbon tetrachloride taken orally will produce acute hepatic necrosis which overshadows the nephrotoxicity. If inhaled, however, renal tubular damage is the dominant problem. Paraquat produces severe ulceration of the oropharynx and leads to a fairly rapid onset of renal failure along with deteriorating respiratory function due to pulmonary fibrosis. The condition is usually irreversible. Ethylene glycol is metabolized to oxalate resulting in a profound systemic acidosis and tubular blockage.

Chapter 21
Congenital and Inherited Abnormalities of the Kidneys and Urinary Tract

Congenital and inherited abnormalities of the urogenital tract occur in about 10% of the population. In some cases these are very minor abnormalities, in others they are significant.

Embryology

Three distinct phases occur in the development of the normal human kidney.

1 The pronephros

This is a rudimentary organ and has no function.

2 The mesonephros

This is functional and develops in association with the Wolffian duct. It develops into a primitive excretory organ with primitive glomeruli and tubules.

3 The metanephros

As the ureteric bud grows from the mesonephric duct, it grows cranially to meet the metanephrogenic cap, which will develop into the metanephros or kidney. The mesonephric tissue at this point atrophies and some of its tubules will remain as part of the excretory apparatus of the testes.

The metanephros develops opposite the third lumbar vertebra, then appears to move in a cephalic direction to lie opposite D 12 L 1. It also rotates medially through 90° so that its pelvis faces medially. Its final blood supply is derived from the dorsal aorta.

Developmental abnormalities, therefore, will result from the following factors.
1   Inadequate renal tissue.

2 Malpositioning of the renal tissue.
3 Malformation of renal tissue.
4 Abnormal differentiation of the tissue.

CONGENITAL DISORDERS

Renal agenesis

Total agenesis is incompatible with extra-uterine life. If it occurs it is often associated with many neuromuscular and skeletal defects. Unilateral agenesis is compatible with normal existence and occurs in approximately 1:1000 of the population, the contralateral kidney being compensatorily hypertrophied.

Renal dysplasia

This is due to disordered development of the renal tissue. The kidney is usually small and irregular and associated abnormalities of the urinary tract may be present. Histologically, dysplastic renal tubules, primitive mesenchymal structures and cysts may be found.

Renal hypoplasia or miniature kidney

In this situation, the renal tissue is normal, though the kidney is extremely small. It is probably due to a deficiency of metanephrogenic tissue during embryological life or to defective branching of the ureteric bud.

With unilateral hypoplasia or dysplasia, compensatory hypertrophy of the contralateral kidney occurs. Both conditions may be associated with hypertension, vesicoureteric reflux and recurrent urinary tract infections.

Ectopic kidneys

These may occur as a result of defective positioning of the metanephrogenic tissue during intra-uterine life. This may result in a pelvically positioned kidney or in both kidneys being positioned on the same side of the vertebral canal—the so-called crossed ectopia (Fig. 21.1). Occasionally both kidneys may be situated in the pelvis.

Urinary infections, obstruction and stone formation may be complications of all these congenital defects.

Pelvic kidneys may interfere with normal parturition and may be
operated upon accidentally (Fig. 21.2).

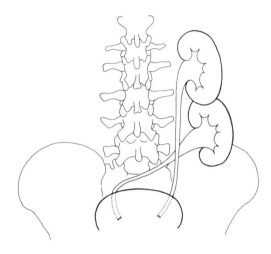

Fig. 21.1   Crossed ectopia.

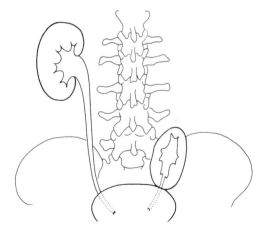

Fig. 21.2   Pelvic kidney.

Horse-shoe kidneys

This is a term to describe kidneys whose lower poles appear to be fused. They are also malrotated. In rare cases the upper poles may also be fused producing a doughnut deformity. Urinary obstruction and stone formation are again complications (Fig. 21.3).

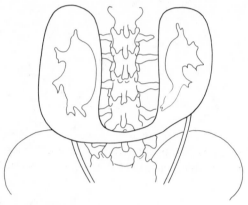

Fig. 21.3 Horse-shoe kidney.

ABNORMALITIES OF THE COLLECTING SYSTEM

Pelvi-ureteric junction (P U J) obstruction

It may be due to either an aberrant branch of the renal artery crossing the pelvi-ureteric junction and therefore distorting it, or disorganization of neuromuscular tissue at the pelvi-uretetic junction. Either condition may produce massive dilatation of the pelvis and calyces, with resulting pain, swelling and infection (Fig. 21.4).

Duplication of the pelvis and ureter

This common abnormality occurs more frequently in females than in males. The ureters on one or both sides may be entirely separated and open independently into the bladder, or they may join with their neighbour at any point from pelvis to bladder. If complete, the upper ureter usually opens at a lower position in the bladder than its

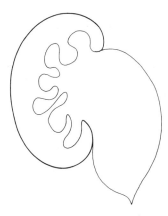

Fig. 21.4   Hydronephrosis due to P U J obstruction.

partner (Fig. 21.5). The position of such ectopic ureters may result in obstruction or incontinence. They are often associated with ureterocoeles.

CONGENITAL ABNORMALITIES OF THE BLADDER AND URETHRA

These abnormalities are usually due to defective development and closure of the ventral structures, often with the result that the pubic rami may remain widely separated.

Prune belly syndrome

This is a condition describing congenital absence of the anterior abdominal wall muscles associated very often with gross dilatation of the ureters and pelvis, dysplastic kidneys and undescended testes (Fig. 21.6).

Ectopia vesicae

Failure of closure of the anterior abdominal structures may result in a spectrum of abnormalities ranging from epispadias (urethral meatus opening on the dorsum of the penis) to complete exposure of the

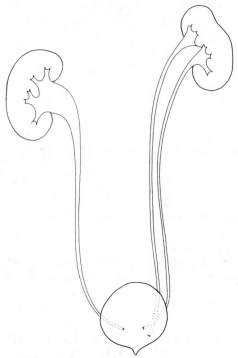

Fig. 21.5   Duplication of pelvis and ureter.

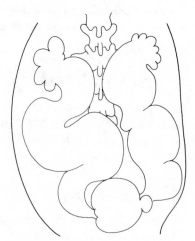

Fig. 21.6   Prune belly syndrome.

bladder. The pubic bones are widely separated. Surgical closure of the abdominal and bladder defect is essential and because the majority of patients will be incontinent, diversion of ureteric urine into an intestinal conduit is usually necessary.

Hypospadias

The external urethral meatus opens on the ventral surface of the penis in the male and in the anterior vaginal wall in the female. Other co-existent anomalies of the upper urinary tract may be present.

Congenital urethral valves

These are flimsy, persistent valve-like structures in the posterior urethra in boys and can quite often cause urinary obstruction. If detected early, they can be destroyed with total restoration of normal bladder function but, if undetected, gross dilatation of the posterior urethra, bladder and ureters can result in permanent renal damage.

CYSTIC DISEASES OF THE KIDNEYS

Various forms of cystic disease can affect the kidneys, ranging from the simple cyst to polycystic disease.

Simple cysts

Simple cysts are usually retention cysts and are seen in the cortex. They are common and are often totally symptom free. Occasionally they grow to a considerable size and cause distortion of the pelvi-calyceal system on that side. They are important from the point of view of being able to distinguish them from renal tumours. This can be achieved by direct cyst puncture under ultrasonic guidance.

Adult polycystic disease

This is a common condition (see Fig. 21.7) which is inherited as an autosomal dominant so that a positive family history of renal disease can usually be obtained. Kidneys usually increase in size gradually, but rarely give symptoms until adult life. It is usually a bilateral condition but rare unilateral cases have been described. Most cases present between the third and fourth decade, the most common symptoms being abdominal distension, pain, recurrent urinary infections, haemorrhage and hypertension. The development of renal stones is not infrequent. Approximately one-third of patients with polycystic kidneys also have cysts in the liver, but these rarely cause problems. The pancreas, lungs, spleen and ovaries may also be cystic. Aneurysms of the Circle of Willis are associated with polycystic disease (approximately 6% of cases) and subarachnoid haemorrhage may be the first indication of cystic disease. Rarely, neoplastic changes can occur in polycystic kidneys.

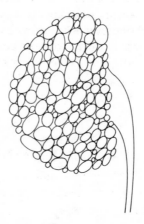

Fig. 21.7 Adult polycystic disease.

Diagnosis

The diagnosis is often made on abdominal examination and can be confirmed by IVU, ultrasound or CT scanning. Haematuria may occur spontaneously, or in association with minor trauma, and patients with polycystic disease usually occupy a prominent place on dialysis and transplant programmes. Owing to a predominantly tubular defect, polyuria and salt wasting may occur and the dangers of dehydration and acidosis are well recognized.

Infantile polycystic disease

Bilateral polycystic disease of infancy is a rare condition occurring in approximately 1:10000 live births. Inheritance is autosomally recessive. Many children with this condition are born dead and obstructive labour may result from the enormous size of the kidneys. If the baby is born alive, it rarely survives long. In those that do survive, hepatic fibrosis leading to portal hypertension may dominate the clinical picture.

Medullary cystic disease

This is a well recognized condition where the kidneys are atrophic with considerable interstitial fibrosis and tubular atrophy. The cysts occur bilaterally and are situated in the corticomedullary region. A familial history is often obtained; it has been described after consanguinous mating and there is a marked association with retinal dysplasia.

The onset of symptoms usually occurs in childhood with anaemia, sodium wasting, loss of urinary concentrating power and progression to chronic renal failure and hypertension.

Multicystic renal dysplasia

This is a common cystic disorder in childhood, usually unilateral or segmental, and presents in early childhood as a renal mass. Cardiac, intestinal and neurological abnormalities may be associated. The cystic changes are probably secondary to dysplastic abnormalities.

Medullary sponge kidneys

This is a non-inherited condition which rarely gives rise to significant trouble though medullary calcification occurs and small stones may be passed with attendant pain and haematuria. Urinary infections are not uncommon. Pyramidal calcification is often seen on the plain film (Fig. 21.8). Characteristic X-ray changes are easily recognized on IVU, for linear shadows radiate outwards from the calyceal cups into the medulla. In the gross section of the kidney the pyramidal medulla appears sponge-like and histologically dilated cystic collect-

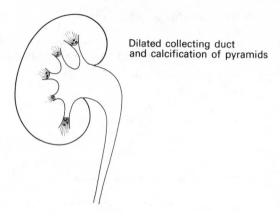

Dilated collecting duct
and calcification of pyramids

Fig. 21.8 Medullary sponge kidney.

ing ducts are seen. The condition may occur in only some or all of the medullary pyramids. The prognosis is excellent, though repeated minor symptoms are often troublesome. Associated skeletal abnormalities have been described, e.g. hemihypertrophy.

Further Reading

ABER G. M. (1982) The kidney in pregnancy. In Jones N. F. & Peters D. K. (eds) *Recent Advances in Renal Medicine 2*. Ch. 10. Churchill Livingstone, London.

ASSCHER A. W., MOFFAT D. B. & SANDERS E. (1982) *Nephrology Illustrated*. Pergamon Medical Publications, Gower Medical Publishing, London.

BECKER LOVEL (ed.) (1977) *Seminars in Nephrology*. John Wiley & Sons, New York.

BERLYNE G. M. (1980) *A Course in Clinical Disorders of Body Fluids and Electrolytes*. Blackwell Scientific Publications, Oxford.

BLACK D. A. K. & JONES N. F. (eds) (1979) *Renal Disease*, 4e. Blackwell Scientific Publications, Oxford.

BOEN S. T. (1961) Kinetics of peritoneal dialysis. A comparison with the artificial kidney. *Medicine (Baltimore)* **40**, 243.

CATTO G. R. D. & SMITH J. A. R. (1981) *Clinical Aspects of Renal Physiology*. Baillière Tindall, London.

CHURG J. & SOKIN L. H. (1982) *Renal Disease. Classification and Atlas of Glomerular Diseases*. Igaku-Shoin, Tokyo.

CURTIS J. R. & WILLIAMS G. B. (1975) *Clinical Management of Chronic Renal Failure*. Blackwell Scientific Publications, Oxford.

DE WARDENER H. E. (1973) *The Kidney*, 4e. J. & A. Churchill Ltd., London.

HAMBURGER J., CROSNIER J. & GRUNFELD J-P. (1979) *Nephrology*. John Wiley & Sons, New York.

IVERSON P. & BRUN C. (1951) Aspiration biopsy of the kidney. *Am. J. Med.* **11**, 324.

JONES N. F. (ed.) (1975) *Recent Advances in Renal Disease*, *I*. Churchill Livingstone, London.

JONES N. F. & PETERS D. K. (eds) (1982) *Recent Advances in Renal Disease*, *II*. Churchill Livingstone, London.

SHERWOOD T. (1980) *Uroradiology*. Blackwell Scientific Publications Ltd., Oxford.

STRAUSS M. B. & WELT L. G. (1979) In Earley L. E. & Gottschalk C. W. (eds) *Diseases of the Kidney*, 3e. Little, Brown & Co., Boston.

TENCKHOFF H. (1974) Peritoneal dialysis today: A new look. *Nephron* **12**, 420.

WARDLE E. N. (1979) *Renal Medicine*. MTP Press.

WILKINSON S. P. (1982) *Hepatorenal Disorders. Kidney Diseases* Vol. 3. Marcel Dekker Inc., New York.

Glossary

ABO	blood groups A, B and O		**DTPA**	diethylenetriamine penta-acetic acid
ACTH	adrenocorticotrophic hormone		**EACA**	epsilon aminocaproic acid
ADH	antidiuretic hormone		**ECF**	extracellular fluid
AMP	adenosine monophosphate		**ECG**	electrocardiogram
ANF	antinuclear factor		**EDTA**	ethylenediamine tetra-acetic acid
ASO	antistreptolysis-O titre		**EM**	electron microscopy
ATN	acute tubular necrosis		**ESR**	erythrocyte sedimentation rate
AV	arteriovenous			
BE	bacterial endocarditis		**FBC**	full blood count
BP	blood pressure			
			GFR	glomerular filtration rate
CA	carbonic anhydrase		**GN**	glomerulonephritis
CAPD	continuous ambulatory peritoneal dialysis			
CCF	congestive heart failure		**HBsAG**	hepatitis B surface antigen
CCI$_4$	carbon tetrachloride		**HLA**	human leucocyte antigens
CHO	carbohydrate			
CIT	cool ischaemic time		**HSP**	Henoch Schönlein purpura
CNS	central nervous system			
CS	Caesarean section		**ICF**	intracellular fluid
CT	computer tomography		**IDH**	ischaemic heart disease
CVP	central venous pressure		**INAH**	isonicotinic acid hydrazide or isoniazid
CYA	cyclosporin A			
			IVC	inferior vena cava
DI	diabetes insipidus		**IVU**	intravenous urogram
DIC	disseminated intravascular coagulation			
			JG	juxtaglomerular
DLE	disseminated or lupus erythematosis		**JVP**	jugular venous pressure
DMSA	dimercaptosuccinic acid			
DMSO	dimethylsulphoxide		**MCGN**	mesangiocapillary glomerulonephritis
DPG	diphosphoglycerate			

6-MP	6-mercaptopurine	**RPF**	retroperitoneal fibrosis
MSU	mid-stream urine	**RTA**	renal tubular acidosis
NG	nasogastric	**SBE**	subacute bacterial endocarditis
PAN	polyarteritis nodosa	**SG**	specific gravity
PAS	para-amino-salicylic acid	**SLE**	systemic lupus erythematosus
PCV	packed cell volume		
PTH	parathyroid hormone	T_3	triiodothyronine
PU	pelvi-ureteric	T_4	thyroxine
PUJ	pelvi-ureteric junction	**TB**	tuberculosis
PUO	pyrexia of unknown origin	**TRH**	thyrotrophin-releasing hormone
		TSH	thyroid-stimulating hormone
QRS	complexes on the ECG	**TTP**	thrombotic thrombocytopenic purpura
RA	rheumatoid arthritis		
rbc	red blood cell (erythrocyte)	**UTI**	urinary tract infections
RES	reticuloendothelial system	**WIT**	warm ischaemia time
RPF	renal plasma flow		

Index